BYPASSING BYPASS

Also by Elmer M. Cranton, M.D.
Trace Elements, Hair Analysis, and Nutrition
(with Richard A. Passwater, Ph.D.)

Also by Arline Brecher
Psychodietetics (with Dr. E. Cheraskin
and Dr. W. M. Ringsdorf)

BYPASSING BYPASS

The New Technique of Chelation Therapy

Elmer M. Cranton, M.D.
and Arline Brecher

Foreword by H. Richard Casdorph, M.D., Ph.D.

STEIN AND DAY/*Publishers*/New York

FIRST STEIN AND DAY PAPERBACK EDITION 1985
Bypassing Bypass was originally published in hardcover by Stein and Day/*Publishers* in 1984.

Designed by Louis A. Ditizio
Printed in the United States of America
STEIN AND DAY/*Publishers*
Scarborough House
Briarcliff Manor, N.Y. 10510
ISBN 0-8128-8183-4

To the members of the American Academy of Medical Preventics and the American Board of Chelation Therapy for the professional contributions to the expansion of human knowledge and the advancement of chelation therapy that they have made

Contents

FOREWORD

In this book Dr. Cranton has taken a quantum step forward in the task of reconciling chelation therapy to traditional medical thinking and understanding. By a series of logical steps, he shows the reader the *meaning* behind the most recent discoveries concerning all forms of degenerative diseases.

Specifically, Dr. Cranton explains the free radical theory of degenerative disease. This new and exciting explanation, which builds upon facts first uncovered in the 1960s, suggests that underlying most degenerative disease—from heart attacks to cancer—is excess free radical activity. If this is the unifying factor behind mankind's major twentieth-century health hazards, then this book will perform the service not merely of demonstrating the merits of an invaluable health care treatment—chelation—but of pinpointing what may be one of the major medical breakthroughs of the century.

For the patient who already has atherosclerosis, the prospect of reversing his disease through chelation treatments is welcome news. It has been shown in experimental animals as well as by blood flow studies in humans that the deposits in arterial walls are reversible. For those people who have not yet begun to feel the effects of atherosclerosis, this book brings home the lessons of preventive medicine. Put very simply, it is wiser to keep one's body in a state of health than to let it deteriorate to a point where a risky surgical procedure such as bypass heart surgery is found advisable.

Bypassing Bypass is a book that will help patients to take responsibility for their own health, and it must be considered required reading for every serious student of preventive medicine—physician and patient alike.

H. Richard Casdorph, M.D., Ph.D.
Assistant Professor of Clinical Medicine,
University of California, Irvine

Introduction

Over 40 million men and women suffer with symptoms of America's number one killer disease. Coronary artery ailments have reached epidemic proportions. One million people die each year. Many are struck down without warning; others succumb after years of painful, debilitating angina—a sure sign that coronary arteries are not delivering enough blood to some area of the heart.

Coronary artery bypass grafting (CABG)—a procedure in which occluded portions of major coronary arteries are bypassed with grafts from a patient's leg veins—is currently the most popular surgical solution to the nation's leading medical problem. Since the procedure was introduced almost two decades ago, both the frequency and the cost of CABGs, or heart bypass operations, as they are commonly called, have escalated. Since 1968, about 1 million heart patients have received this surgical treatment. In 1976, about 80,000 patients with an average bill of $12,000 underwent surgical coronary artery "repair." In 1981, close to 160,000 were operated on and the per-patient cost rose to approximately $20,000. Nearly 200,000 such operations were performed in 1983—$25,000 to $40,000 bills were common. Bypass surgery has grown to a $3 billion a year industry.

Reasonable men and women might logically assume the runaway popularity of this enthusiastically prescribed treatment has been based on convincing and demonstrable evidence that it prolongs life—or at least, has the potential to prevent further health deterioration. If that were indeed true, there would be far less need for me to write—or you to read—this book.

As things actually stand, professional enthusiasm for the operation can scarcely be justified by patient outcomes. A ten-year, $24 million study conducted by the National Heart, Lung and Blood Institute, which screened 16,000 patients (with persistent angina but without severe obstruction of the left anterior descending coronary artery) who underwent CABGs at 11 leading medical centers, revealed no increase in post-surgical survival rates as compared with a matched group of nonsurgically treated patients. As for quality of life, again no difference between the two groups: they were on a par when it came to employment and recreational status.

A good case against rushing into bypass surgery is made by the study, released in 1983, which concluded that at least one out of every seven patients might have safely postponed his operation or avoided it altogether. Approximately 25,000 operations each year were unnecessary, the researchers said, noting that in many cases it might be more judicious to delay surgery than not. Bypass surgery does not cure the underlying disease and may indeed actually induce its more rapid progression. One thing the general public is not fully aware of is that many people need a *second* bypass. Sometimes the blood vessels that weren't bypassed become clogged and need bypassing; sometimes the transplanted vessels used in the first graft run into the same trouble; sometimes the transplants malfunction or turn out to be too small for the job. Once you've had a bypass, your chances of needing another go up about 5 percent a year. Research shows that ten years after surgery, grafted vessels had closed in 40 percent of patients, and in the remaining 60 percent, half developed further coronary artery narrowing.

No discussion of the pros and cons of CABG would be complete without mentioning the physical and emotional trauma associated with bypass, or the risks involved. In one to four percent of the cases, depending on the medical center and the surgical team, surgery is fatal, and in up to five percent, the surgery itself precipitates a heart attack. In 20 percent of the cases serious—sometimes permanent—personality changes result (forgetfulness, irritability, insomnia, inability to concentrate, mental confusion). This seldom mentioned aftereffect, thought to be caused by tiny air bubbles entering the brain from the external blood pump used while the heart is stopped, happens commonly enough that when one California cardiovascular surgeon had to undergo bypass surgery himself, he arranged to spend several hours immediately before and after surgery in the hospital's hyperbaric oxygen unit, hoping to reduce his risk of brain damage. There was only one hospital in his region of California that had a hyperbaric chamber, and this surgeon had enough pull to see to it that he was operated on there.

Even if bypass technology were perfected to the point where every procedure were a resounding success (no one suffered, no one died from surgical complications, grafts remained unoccluded), legitimate questions could still be raised concerning the surgery's validity.

How can such a piecemeal surgical "cure" be worthwhile? What lasting benefit can result from a procedure that detours a few impaired arteries while many others throughout the body continue to deteriorate? There is an inherent fallacy in bypassing only one or even several restricted portions of the body's blood vessels, when the same degenerating condition must be affecting the entire cardiovascular system. The bypass approach treats the tip of the iceberg—the sites where plaque has developed most rapidly—while ignoring the rest of the circulatory network. At best, it is an expensive stopgap measure, a risky, high-priced surgical "aspirin," providing pain relief and not much more.

The fact that most CABG patients do experience a reduction of pain—that many are angina-free for two to five years—may be more of a minus than a plus, since the absence of chest pain may encourage them to believe themselves medically improved. The patient who thinks himself restored to health when he is not may well return to his former unhealthy lifestyle, not realizing he is still in jeopardy.

With all the publicity given to its risks and drawbacks, why do so many continue to opt for the bypass operation?

The answer: Atherosclerotic patients have been misled into expecting better results than objective statistics warrant and they are rarely offered alternatives.

"What choice did I have?" is a common patient comment. "My doctor had nothing else to suggest."

Arterial dilating drugs such as nitroglycerin work for some for a time; blood thinners can cause as big a problem as they correct; the newer medications such as beta-blockers and calcium antagonists are effective but have not proved universally useful; for those in great pain, or facing imminent heart failure, stringent exercise and diet regimens take too long; balloon angioplasty, laser therapy, and metal coil artery reaming are all promising, but still experimental.

And the most worthy alternative—chelation therapy—is almost never mentioned.

Chelation therapy is a medical treatment that improves metabolic and circulatory function by removing toxic metals (such as lead and cadmium) and abnormally located nutritional metallic ions (such as copper and iron) from the body. This is accomplished by administering a synthetic amino acid, ethylene-diamine-tetra-acetic acid (EDTA), by an intravenous infusion using a tiny 25-gauge needle.

An informal survey of well-read followers of the latest health news revealed that few had heard of chelation therapy; fewer still had more than a vague idea of what it is. In those rare instances where an individual knew that chelation therapy offers a safe and effective alternative to bypass surgery, he or she had "stumbled" across the information accidentally—a friend or relative had been successfully chelated—and had passed the word along. Chelation therapy may be this decade's best kept medical secret. In recent years almost as many patients are being chelated as bypassed, in most cases with superior results.

Thus the real reason for this book extends far beyond the overuse or abuse of bypass surgery. The fact is that a major therapy (chelation), which offers a greatly improved quality of life for millions of people *with many different age-related diseases*, has been overlooked and is being suppressed and discriminated against by the medical profession.

The disservice to the public cannot be overestimated. Chelation therapy has shown itself to be of value in an incredible variety of supposedly incurable diseases in a significant percentage of patients. While it is true that physicians who practice chelation have not yet been able to put together the hard data to substantiate the long-term health benefits to patients suffering from degenerative diseases of all types, that does not discredit chelation. Chelating physicians are private practitioners with limited resources, unable to fund the large-scale, well-designed and scientifically irrefutable double-blind studies that impress the medical community. Properly done, such research would without doubt confirm clinical impressions and smaller studies that have demonstrated the extraordinary value of this treatment.

Why has funding been so hard to come by? Perhaps the pervasive anti-chelation stance is easier to understand with the knowledge that chelation therapy does not require the vast resources of modern medical centers. It makes no use of the full panoply of space-age technology so prominent at research-oriented hospitals. While there is nothing about chelation that smacks of wizardry or quackery (it cannot be administered by anyone other than a fully licensed medical doctor) it can be done in a clinician's office on an outpatient basis. That is a benefit to patients but a decided drawback to funding. There can be no profit in proving the validity of chelation therapy to those who most influence funding decisions.

Chelation therapy is nonsurgical and requires only a series of visits (several hours each) to a physician's treatment facilities for the intravenous infusion of an FDA-approved medicine, the synthetic amino acid EDTA (ethylene-diamine-tetra-acetic acid). Although EDTA has little effect on cholesterol or triglycerides in the arterial plaque, it does disrupt the disease process in ways to be explained later. The effects of treatment can be dramatic in a short period of time. Often, patients who could not walk across the floor without taking nitroglycerin for their angina pains are out playing golf in a matter of six to eight weeks.

The seemingly miraculous, "too good to be true" flavor of many of the testimonials to chelation therapy's benefits have hindered, rather than helped, its acceptance. No wonder. Medical scientists have only recently begun to comprehend the interrelationship of many apparently unconnected ailments. Chelating physicians have been embarrassed, rather than pleased, to have patients report improvement of symptoms of a whole host of diseases, including arthritis, multiple sclerosis, Parkinson's disease, and psoriasis, when they could not explain the reasons behind their recovery. Such cures have been considered so outlandishly improbable that rumors regarding them have only served to cast further doubts on the credibility of chelation's proponents.

But science is beginning to make good sense out of what has been a bad joke. The very latest buzz words in scientific circles are "free radical pathology." Scientists in laboratories in all parts of the world are agog over the discovery that there is a common denominator among many degenerative diseases—atherosclerosis, included—and that this common denominator is a disease mechanism called free radical pathology (a process you'll be hearing a great deal more about), which comes about by virtue of the production in our bodies of a form of oxygen that in its unstable state is called super oxide and hydroxyl radicals, peroxide, and singlet oxygen.

What happens is that oxygen "goes wrong" in the body at certain points and under certain conditions and this excited form of oxygen reacts with literally anything nearby, causing damage to tissues and cells akin to radiation exposure.

In contrast to surgical and other medical modalities, chelation therapy counteracts the underlying disease process. Once in the bloodstream, intravenous injections of EDTA block excess free radical production, protecting the tissues and organs from further damage. Over time, these injections halt the progress of the free radical disease that is the underlying condition triggering the development of atherosclerosis (and other degenerative conditions). They give the body time to heal, and they restore adequate blood flow through occluded arteries so as to relieve symptoms of arterial insufficiency in every part of the body.

Unlike the surgical approach that, in effect, pretends vascular disease is a segmented localized ailment, chelation theory recognizes that the condition affects not only individual arteries, such as the coronaries around the heart, but also the arteries to every organ in the body and the tiniest arterioles and capillaries in toes and fingers. Sixty thousand people per year lose legs from gangrene caused by arterial blockages. Many more than that have strokes. Bypass surgeries to arteries in the legs, neck, and even inside the skull is quite common.

Even if you are at this moment symptom-free—with no indication that plaque is insidiously accumulating in your arteries, gradually reducing life-preserving cardiovascular circulation—you nonetheless suffer some degree of free radical pathology. The slow breakdown of biochemical efficiency that inexorably leads to interference with the body's structure and functions starts in infancy and becomes increasingly debilitating over time, depending on inherited resiliency, environmental exposure, and current lifestyle.

Unless you embrace a program of health-promoting strategies designed to stall off biological deterioration, you are sure to develop some form of free radical disease—diabetes, arthritis, Parkinson's, Alzheimer's, atherosclerosis, cancer, to name just a few—ailments mistakenly thought to be the inescapable consequences of so-called "normal aging." When the breakdown comes, you may well find yourself in a crisis-care predicament, faced with a treatment-decision dilemma. Under the urgency of the moment, chances are slim you would ever be offered the "chelation option."

Prior to this book, you would have to be extremely lucky to know such an option even exists. That is not apt to be true much longer. Now that there is growing recognition of the free radical processes in human disease, the next step will be the scurry to develop new forms of treatment to combat free radical damage. Without doubt, scientists will soon discover—much to their astonishment, of course—that a large portion of current treatments with drugs and diets that have proven effective already depend on free radical mechanisms. Scientists who once scoffed at the therapeutic benefits of nutrients such as Vitamin C, Vitamin E, selenium, manganese, and zinc are apt to rethink their position in light of the proven biological anti-oxidant properties of these substances.

And those who have been so eager to deride chelation without ever having taken a serious look at it are going to be hardput to uphold their anti-chelation bias now that it is clear that chelation therapy is the granddaddy of all anti-free radical treatments. Chelation is the already available, remarkable, life-prolonging treatment that reverses the symptoms of not only atherosclerosis but almost all other age-related degenerative diseases.

BYPASSING BYPASS

1

Chelation? It Must Be Something New!

"Chelation? It must be something new."
Why do you say that?
"I never heard of it."
So?
"It couldn't be any good."
Why?
"Good news spreads fast!"

"Chelation? That doesn't work."
Why do you say that?
"It's been around for years."
So?
"It couldn't be any good."
Why?
"It would be popular by now!"

Objections to chelation on either grounds are unfounded. The truth is that chelation therapy is both old and new.

The history of chelation therapy can be traced back to 1893 and the pioneering research of Swiss Nobel laureate Alfred Werner, who developed the theories that later became the foundation of modern chelation chemistry. Werner's concept of how metals bind to organic molecules opened the new field of chelation chemistry.

It was not until the early 1920s that "chelation" was introduced as an industrial tool, finding wide application in the manufacture of paint, rubber, and petroleum. Chelation was also found to be useful in the separation of specific metals, and it gained importance in electroplating and industrial dye manufacture.

In the mid-1930s, German industrialists, concerned with their reliance on imports from potentially unfriendly countries, embarked on a major effort to develop their own chelating agents. Citric acid, a chelating compound used for stain prevention in the printing of textiles, was high on their substitution list.

Their mission: to develop a synthetic calcium-binding additive to keep stains from forming when calcium in hard water reacted with certain dyes. The substance developed—ethylene-diamine-tetra-acetate, or EDTA, as it is commonly known—was patented in 1935. EDTA proved to be more successful than anticipated. It was both effective and inexpensive, superior in many ways to the citric acid it replaced.

In the years that followed, EDTA synthesis was further refined and modified both in Germany and in the United States. Marketed under many trade names, EDTA's commercial uses expanded as researchers perfected its ability to leech heavy metals, such as lead, from biological and chemical systems.

Today EDTA and other chelators are in homes as well as factories—in hundreds of everyday products. Few consumers realize that were it not for the chelating effects of household detergents, dirtied wash water would not drain free of scum. There would be an unsightly residue left around wash basins and tubs.

For all its industrial success, it was not until World War II that the potential therapeutic benefits of chelation were realized. Government concern with the possibility of poison gas warfare triggered a mammoth search for suitable antidotes.

The search ended when a team of English researchers, headed by Professor R. A. Peters at Oxford, implemented the chelation principle using BAL (British Anti-Lewisite, a chelating compound), which rendered arsenic from poison gases less harmful.

At the end of the war, chelation therapy was introduced into the medical arena. During the 1940s it became the routine treatment for arsenic and other metal poisonings. Poison gas fears proved to be unfounded, but a far graver public threat was developing: the real possibility of radioactive fallout that might contaminate mass populations should the atom bomb, then a hush-hush project, become a reality. Most radioactive contamination is in the form of isotopes of metallic ions, which can be chelated.

Americans, fortunately, were spared both eventualities, and the therapeutic use of chelation did not cross the ocean until the early 1950s. A group of workers suffering lead poisoning in a battery factory in Michigan were successfully detoxified. The chelating agent used was EDTA, found by American scientists to be more effective with fewer adverse side effects than the British compound.

Next, the U.S. Navy adopted EDTA chelation therapy for sailors who had absorbed lead while painting ships and other naval facilities. By the mid-1950s, it was the accepted "treatment of choice" for lead poisoning in children and adults and, as of today, it still is.

The first indication of EDTA chelation therapy's potential for conditions other than lead poisoning surfaced when chelated persons reported surprising post-chelation health improvements—better memory, vision, hearing, and sense of smell, and clearer thinking—all seemingly unrelated to lead removal.

More to the point, patients suffering from atherosclerosis in addition to lead poisoning reported surprising post-chelation rewards: They were able to walk farther, with less chest or leg pain. Those with angina were able to exert themselves without discomfort. They tired less easily and had much improved physical endurance.

Such dramatic benefits, chelating physicians theorized, could not possibly be explained simply by the removal of lead; they had to be related in some way to increased blood flow through or around blocked arteries.

Intrigued by these new developments, cardiologists began to investigate and research the possibilities of chelation as a therapy for circulatory ailments, atherosclerosis, and related disorders. Early findings were encouraging and duly reported in the American medical literature beginning in the early 1950s.

Two of the earliest researchers were Dr. Albert J. Boyle, professor of chemistry at Wayne State University in Detroit, and Dr. Gordon B. Myers, professor of medicine at the same university and one of the best-known cardiologists of his day.

Working at Providence Hospital in Detroit, they took on the "basket cases"—people so incapacitated by atherosclerotic cardiovascular disease that they were considered beyond help. And those patients improved. Two such individuals had damaged heart valves, generally understood to be an incurable condition without open heart surgery. Following chelation these and other patients enjoyed a remarkable return of cardiac function and a reversal of disabling symptoms.

Clinical studies continued, and published reports consistently described identifiable signs of improved coronary circulation and heart function in most atherosclerotic patients after chelation. The findings—that patients had improved skin color, a return of normal temperature to cold extremities, improved muscular coordination and brain function, improved exercise tolerance without angina or shortness of breath, and a reduced need for pain relievers—were duly published in the scientific journals. There have been dozens of such published clinical reports to date.

By 1964 the world's medical literature contained numerous scientific observations confirming the early findings. In that year, the distinguished Alfred Soffer, M.D., associate in medicine at Northwestern University Medical School and the former director of the Cardiopulmonary Laboratory of Rochester, New York, writing in his book, *Chelation Therapy,* stated that atherosclerotic patients suffering from occlusive peripheral vascular disease appeared to benefit from repeated administration of EDTA, especially those patients with diabetes.

A great deal of progress has since been made in the clinical use of EDTA chelation therapy for atherosclerosis.

Clinical trials testing the effectiveness of EDTA chelation therapy in the treatment of arterial occlusion continue. Two of the most recent were performed by H. Richard Casdorph, M.D., Ph.D., assistant clinical professor of medicine at the University of California Medical School in Irvine, and by Drs. E. W. McDonagh, C. J. Rudolph, and E. Cheraskin.

All three studies demonstrate statistically significant increases in blood flow following treatment. Objective measurements were made before and after EDTA chelation therapy, using individual patients as their own controls.

Dr. Casdorph, utilizing sophisticated new noninvasive radioactive isotopes, demonstrated a highly significant improvement of heart function and a highly significant increase in blood flow to the brain in patients with atherosclerosis. Precise measurements of cardiac ejection fraction (the percentage of blood pumped from the large chamber of the heart with each contraction) was determined before and after chelation therapy. Similar techniques were used to measure blood flow in carotid arteries leading to the brain and through the brain itself. The statistical probabilities that measured improvement could have been due to pure chance were less than one in ten thousand.

Dr. McDonagh and his colleagues in Kansas duplicated the Casdorph brain blood flow study results using a different technique. By varying pressure on an eyeball, it is possible to determine the pressure of arterial blood flow to the back of the eye. Since the eye and the brain are physiologically integrated, the eye reflects brain circulation.

Patients were used as their own controls, with measurements taken before and after chelation therapy. Improvements were also found by McDonagh to be highly significant.

These two excellent studies of blood flow to the brain were performed independently by different researchers in different locations, using different measurement techniques. The scientific community traditionally accepts the results of important new findings when results have been independently confirmed by separate researchers in unaffiliated facilities. These two independent studies followed scientific protocol, demonstrated a measurable effect of EDTA chelation therapy (increased blood flow to the brain) and served to substantiate what individual chelating physicians have observed independently.

Even without such sophisticated tests, we could presume that there was increased blood flow by sight and by touch. Patients routinely get their color back; their once-pasty complexions develop a healthy glow. Cold limbs regain warmth. Icy toes and icy fingers heat up. All this in addition to a dramatic reduction of symptoms resulting from diminished blood flow.

Clinical results are invariably impressive. In the majority of cases, patients suffering the catastrophic effects of atherosclerosis (coronary artery disease, blockage of arteries to the brain causing stroke and senility, high blood pressure, peripheral vascular blockage of arteries to the legs, early gangrene, various types of arthritic and other related disorders) experience improved health. They regain physical and mental functions. They begin to "live" again.

As of this writing, more than 400,000 patients have received in excess of 6 million chelation treatments in the United States alone, and without a single proven fatality caused by chelation when the treatment was properly administered and supervised.

If the reader is mystified at this point, no wonder.

If chelation therapy is not old and discredited—and not new and untried—then what is going on?

If a safe, effective, tested, legal, nonsurgical treatment that seems able to reverse the symptoms of atherosclerosis and improve blood flow exists, then why haven't you heard of it?

2

The Making of a Chelation Doctor

I did not set out to be a chelation doctor—or any kind of medical specialist, for that matter. After completing training at Harvard Medical School, all I wanted was a traditional family practice. No fancy surgery, no Nobel prize-winning research, not even a six-figure income and four cars in the garage.

Ambitions? Sure. I hoped to find a nice town where I could be Dr. Welby to whole families, treating all kinds of everyday ailments and complaints.

After some years as a naval flight surgeon, I spent six years as a family practitioner in southern California in group practice. And then, while in Los Angeles attending a medical meeting in mid-1972, I heard a tale that was to change my life. It began with an innocent enough invitation.

"If you're not busy after dinner, drop into Room 1272."

"What's up?"

"George wants to tell just a few of us about something new he's stumbled on—it's pretty revolutionary."

I was quick to accept, for the "George" referred to was—and still is—an eminent and respected physician, a board-certified ear, nose, and throat specialist, and chief of otolaryngology at two hospitals. If "George" had something to report, I wanted to hear it.

"In case you're wondering," our host began later that same evening, "what you've heard was correct. I did suffer a severe angina attack last year and was warned of the imminent danger of a ardial infarct. As a matter of fact, a few Long Beach doctors are rprised I'm still alive.

"As you can see, I'm back at work full time, and feeling a hell of a lot better than anyone, including myself, would have thought possible six months ago. The way that came about is what I want to tell you about."

Like all too many victims of advanced atherosclerosis, George first knew he was seriously ill when he was suddenly seized with severe chest pains.

As he told it: "There I was, enjoying a round of golf, when all at once, I felt as though an elephant had jumped on my chest."

The doctor became a patient. All the appropriate diagnostic procedures were performed at one of the nation's top medical schools: electrocardiograms, treadmill tests, a coronary angiogram, the works. The results were not consoling.

Doctors level with one another.

"It doesn't look good, George," the cardiologists said, reporting the angiogram had revealed plaque blockages obstructing the left main coronary artery, and other arteries as well. Their recommendation was a triple coronary artery bypass.

"No time to waste," the specialists agreed, pointing out there was impending danger of total occlusion, and a real possibility of sudden death.

"Ouch," George said.

Physicians are as apprehensive as laymen when it comes to going "under the knife"—perhaps more so, being all too familiar with what can go wrong with major surgery.

Coronary artery bypass is a particularly sobering prospect, inasmuch as it entails any number of hazards. During the 1970s, a significant percentage of patients—as high as 10 to 15 percent—died as a direct result of the surgery. Survivors had no assurance of long-term improvement. No one could say for sure that the bypassed arteries would not degenerate further, or that new occlusions might not develop at the site of the graft. It was a high-risk surgical procedure with uncertain benefits. Today the procedures have been improved and a lot fewer people die on the operating table, but the benefits are still uncertain.

For George, however, there did not seem to be any choice. Then fate intervened.

The Christmas holidays were looming, and the Red Cross was unable to supply the seven standby units of blood required until after New Year's. George chose not to remain idle during his two-week reprieve.

"I talked about my condition to everybody I could get hold of—doctors, lawyers, my golfing buddies, my accountant."

A week later, a physician George described as "a very dear colleague who went to medical school with me, interned with me, and later became a prominent New York internist," called to ask, "Ever heard of chelation?"

"How do you spell it?" George asked, and headed for the medical library.

"I'm sure you fellows are going to be as amazed as I was," he told us. "There are a couple dozen or so pretty impressive clinical reports on this chelation therapy that I'll bet most of you have never heard of."

Further investigation led to a decision to postpone surgery long enough to give this apparently safe, painless, noninvasive therapy a chance to work. Intent on being treated by a doctor experienced in chelation, George traveled more than 2,000 miles to one of the few clinics in the country then specializing in the treatment.

"You're going to find the rest of this hard to believe," he warned.

"After only ten of those treatments, my angina disappeared—completely! Imagine how I felt. Before I started treatment, I couldn't walk a dozen steps without severe angina. But, I swear, I haven't had a chest pain since.

"What's more, I saw dozens of other patients, even worse off than myself, healed from conditions you and I know are incurable. One arrived with a gangrenous leg, and I saw that man's leg return to normal.

"Some of the things I saw made me wonder if I could believe my own eyes: people checked in with chronic diabetic ulcerative lesions and gangrenous lesions that began normal healing in ten to twelve days."

Ordinarily somewhat reserved, George waxed on with uncharacteristic enthusiasm, crediting chelation with astonishing cures, not the least of which was his own.

"I carry a full work load. I do approximately ten to fifteen surgeries every week, and these are microsurgeries of the ear. I carry a full practice. I play golf. I swim 20 laps in my pool every day, and I cannot speak with any but the greatest praise for the men who are attempting to make chelation an accepted form of therapy."

If it were anyone but George reporting such wonders, I doubt that any of the physicians listening, myself included, would have given much credence to so fanciful a tale. But it was impossible to doubt his sincerity, integrity, and even more important, his medical credibility.

We had dozens of questions:

"What did the treatment involve?"

A series of intravenous injections.

"How many treatments—how long?"

George had taken a series of 20 treatments, each taking three to four hours, at the clinic, and had since learned to self-administer the intravenous injections with the help of a nurse at home.

"Was it legal?"

"Yes."

"Was it painful?"

"No."

"Was it safe?"

"Yes."

"Did it work in every case?"

"What does?"

"Why haven't we heard about it before?"

The key question.

George did not have a good answer.

Chelation therapy has been relegated to a medical no man's land ever since the chelating agent—EDTA—which had formerly been accepted by the Food and Drug Administration (FDA) for the treatment of occlusive vascular diseases (such as angina) lost this status because of an unfortunate, uncontested change in Federal regulations.

Previously it had only been necessary to prove EDTA's safety. That was no problem. To meet the newly regulated FDA requirement for proof of effectiveness for the treatment of atherosclerosis would require that tens of millions of dollars be spent on research. No drug company was willing to underwrite such an expense because the patent on the substance had already expired. And there was no longer hope for recovery of costs.

Chelation with EDTA was—and still is—the FDA-accepted treatment for lead poisoning and dangerously high blood calcium, but physicians electing to use the treatment for any other purpose do so at the risk of flouting FDA guidelines and the recommendation of the American Medical Association. While a physician may legally use any FDA-approved drug however he deems suitable, he does risk increased vulnerability to malpractice suits (and the frowns of his colleagues) when he defies established recommendations.

George was optimistic that EDTA chelation therapy for atherosclerosis could not remain in limbo for long.

"It's too good to be ignored," he said. "All that's needed is for a reputable group of physicians to get moving on this—to study up, start treating patients, and document its value."

George made it clear that he hoped there were doctors among the group invited to witness his testimony who would "get the chelation ball rolling." It was an irresistible challenge. Even if George were not so well respected, we would have been eager to find out whether chelation therapy would hold up to more intensive scrutiny.

It was a lucky time for anyone interested in a novel medical modality to be practicing in California, where so many new ideas—political, social, and scientific—seem to take root and grow. The informal study group of about a dozen doctors that formed that night (and eventually spawned the American Academy of Medical Preventics and the American Board of Chelation Therapy) began meeting regularly. There were seminars, lectures, and physician training sessions. Doctors learned to improve chelation techniques by apprenticing to each other.

The more I learned, the more intrigued I became. I read dozens of monographs and hundreds of articles in various medical journals published here and abroad. I talked at length to pioneer chelation practitioners, and interviewed many of their patients. I signed on for courses and learned to administer the therapy. I shared experiences with colleagues doing the same, and all of us agreed that chelation therapy was so worthwhile, it would soon be a universally accepted and practiced treatment.

That was in 1972. It hasn't happened yet. As it turns out, George is an astute scientist, but a rotten prophet.

I chose to leave the scene for a brief time, when my long-standing involvement with public health and preventive medicine led to a position with the U.S. Public Health Service. I became Chief-of-Staff at the Talihina, Oklahoma, Indian Hospital, where I supervised the medical care of 12,000 Choctaw. Although that assignment removed me from active involvement with chelation, my interest never dimmed. During that stint, I kept in touch with chelation practitioners, stayed current with the new literature, and took annual refresher courses. Finally, in 1976, it seemed the right time to settle down somewhere with my wife, Nancy, and our four young children.

Through the medical grapevine I heard of an opportunity to set up a full-time family practice in a small town, Trout Dale, in southwestern Virginia's Blue Ridge Mountains. The Mount Rogers Clinic (a modern out-patient facility) was to be my headquarters, and I would be the only doctor within a 20-mile radius.

Trout Dale (population 250 but with 4000 people residing within ten miles of my office) isn't really "near" anywhere. It is more than an hour and a half drive to the closest big city, and the nearest movie and supermarket is 35 minutes away by car. I was not just a family doctor, now; I was a country doctor.

Some days were frantic; others were not. Sometimes I worked round the clock; other times I could have gone fishing and no one would have noticed. I was on call 24 hours a day, seven days a week. The Mount Rogers Clinic was not only my office but my home as well, providing living quarters for my family. Oh yes, we were also the local pharmacy.

It was the perfect setting for my one-on-one, prevention-minded brand of medicine. I am a holistically oriented doctor—a maverick in the eyes of some of my colleagues. I use whatever treatments work best for my patients, even if not yet endorsed by the more conservative medical groups. For example, I have long advised dietary changes and vitamin supplementation to enhance other remedies. Long before it was popular, I was encouraging patients to exercise regularly and to upgrade their nutrition.

At first, my medical practice focused mainly on the routine: ear infections, broken arms, pneumonia, and gout. There was the occasional car wreck, accidental poisoning, serious burn, personal assault injury, on-the-job accident, or other medical trauma. It made for a full life—a typical quiet, country doctor existence—until I introduced chelation therapy.

Rural Virginians develop vascular diseases just like big city folk, and they are no more eager than their urban counterparts to undergo surgery. One of the first patients I chelated was a wealthy businessman whose heart specialist had told him, "Get your affairs in order. You won't last long."

When after a full course of treatments, he was back at work, putting in an eight-hour day, acting 20 years younger, we lost our Walton Mountain-style seclusion forever. On the basis of initial successes, patients sent others, many far from Trout Dale. Our daily caseload soon included men and women from up and down the eastern seaboard. Like born again evangelists, our recovered chelation patients regarded it as their mission to spread the word.

And for good reason. Many consider their cure nothing short of a miracle. Detailed case histories time and again document remarkable recoveries from an almost endless variety of so-called hopeless degenerative ailments.

Chelation therapy is not a cure-all or an "elixir of life," but it can do things that no other therapy or surgical procedure presently available has any hope of achieving. The next chapter is an illustration of that fact.

3

The Story of J.

She came to my clinic in rural Virginia in April of 1979. J. had nowhere else to go, and she was in dreadful—almost terminal—shape.

Like many of my patients, J. had rejected the advice of her physician to undergo immediate surgery. She had developed gangrene in her right foot and was advised to have it amputated. J. was not quite 50 years old, a working woman, and a grandmother. She had suffered with increasing poor circulation caused by atherosclerosis for a good many years. She had lived by her wits all her life, and she was determined not to lose one of her limbs—even if she had to die to keep it. So she came to me.

According to most cardiovascular surgeons and specialists, there is only one remedy for a limb becoming blackened with gangrene resulting from end-stage atherosclerosis: cut it off before it poisons the whole body.

I do not accept that in every case. Especially where the gangrene has just begun, chelation therapy can often restore blood circulation and promote healing.

Amputation, on the other hand, neither treats nor eliminates the root cause of ischemic gangrene (blocked circulation and oxygen starvation), which will most likely recur at a future time higher up in the severed limb or in the other leg.

Rather than remove the gangrenous leg, I prefer to try chelation, not just because this is a less mutilating approach to a devastating ailment, but because it allows more options. If successful, the limb will be restored to normal, or at least acceptable functioning. Minor surgery may be needed to trim away the dead tissue only. If chelation should prove unsuccessful, amputation is still available as a last resort.

In J's case, ischemic gangrene had surfaced in her right foot, which had begun ulcerating three months before. Soon the foot was mottled with black patches. Three toes, then the heel, developed festering wounds that oozed a dark, smelly discharge. J.'s pain throbbed unceasingly, making it impossible for her to work, walk, even to sleep.

Attending doctors offered J. a Hobson's choice: your foot or your life. But J. would have none of it. She suspected the first excision would most likely lead to another. And another. Her atherosclerotic wounds evidenced a progressive disease.

"I am not going to have any more surgery," J. resolved. "If the pain gets *too* bad, I'll blow my brains out."

J.'s decision resulted from a long and expensive medical history that had left her physically and emotionally scarred. After filing for bankruptcy, because of huge medical bills, she had had her fill of hospitals and operations and doctors, however well intentioned their advice. For a solid year, since March 1978, J.'s life had entailed a grueling series of expensive, unproductive medical consultations and confinements. Despite everything, her health had continued to deteriorate.

She could hardly recall a time when she could get around pain-free. For years, whenever she climbed stairs, took a walk, or stood in line, she would experience leg cramps and throbbing pain. "When I complained to doctors, they would tell me, 'Don't worry. It's all in your mind.'" The pains in J.'s legs continually grew worse.

"Then came the day my body finally gave out. I just collapsed." When J. came to, she was in intensive care at DePaul Hospital in Norfolk, Virginia. Her left side was numb and it was thought she had developed embolisms, small blood clots or tiny pieces of atherosclerotic plaque that break off from an arterial wall and circulate through the bloodstream until they become lodged in the narrow, downstream segments of blood vessels. Three angiograms were performed. "A ghastly experience," J. recalls.

The diagnosis was grave: total occlusion of the left subclavian artery, and far-advanced blockage of the arterial systems to her left arm and right leg. Translated, J. had end-stage hardening of the arteries—critical blood vessel blockages that severely limited circulation throughout her body and especially to her extremities.

Then, as now, the commonly accepted surgical treatment for J.'s ailment was arterial surgery. There were three operations in J.'s case: the first, to replace the descending aorta and iliac arteries with a man-made "Y" graft; the second to bypass the blockage in her right leg; and the last for the left arm. Assured that there was no alternative, J. reluctantly agreed to the first operation.

"It almost killed me," she reports. "I went into cardiac arrest twice."

After that ordeal, J. was too weak for further surgery. She was discharged from Norfolk Hospital, prognosis "improved" but still suffering from occlusive peripheral vascular disease, a threatening condition that inevitably deteriorates. In J.'s case, it wasn't long before she knew she was destined for more trouble. Her pains were as bad as ever. The surgery had brought no relief at all. The branch of arterial "Y" graft leading to her right leg had blocked off once again.

"The slightest activity was a pain-filled huff and puff effort," J. remembers. "I felt I was living on borrowed time. I stopped making plans more than one week ahead."

She maintained her regular medical checkups. "Each time I questioned my doctors about what to do next, the answer was always the same: 'More surgery.'"

At this time, the late autumn of 1978, J. was truly desperate for some alleviation of her disabling pain, any kind of alternative to the dreaded arterial surgery. As it happened, our paths crossed. I was the featured speaker at a holistic health seminar in Roanoke. J. was there and she buttonholed me in the parking lot.

I could see right away how distraught she was, how frantically she wanted an empathetic listener. J. rattled off her medical history, and expressed interest in my talk about the healthful benefits of diet, exercise, and vitamin supplements. But what had really caught her attention had been my brief remarks about chelation therapy and its effectiveness in reversing the symptoms of atherosclerosis.

"I've never heard of chelation," she said. She wanted to find out more. I mailed her an information packet. She wrote back saying she did not think she could afford any more regular medical care.

"Your clinic in Trout Dale," she explained "might just as well be in another country as four hours away. I'm broke, depressed, and have run out of health insurance. Constant illness has forced me to change jobs a lot and lose benefits. And I still owe for old medical bills. It hardly seems the time to take leave from my job again."

But in January 1979, J. was forced to rearrange her priorities once more, and put survival at the top of the list.

"I began to suspect it was the beginning of the end," she remembered. What triggered her presentiment was a sore big toe, a very sore big toe, which refused to get better. "I tried all the usual treatments, but it just got blacker and wouldn't heal.

"Then, the toe began to seep. And ooze. I had been swimming a lot, but I gave it up because I was afraid that whatever I had might be contagious. Then the rest of the foot began to ache and look funny." It was time for J. to see a doctor again.

Her worst fears were confirmed. The arterial graft in her right leg had completely blocked. Almost all circulation to the foot was gone and ischemic gangrene had set in. The consulting surgeon did not mince words: amputate right now, just below the knee, and stay alive.

"More surgery? Never. No way," J. replied.

The surgeon shrugged, as much as to say, "It's your funeral."

And J. was resigned to her fate. Her condition worsened with each passing day. She could no longer walk; she had to be carried upstairs where she worked, then hobble painfully to her desk. "It all seemed so hopeless," she recalls. "I was fully prepared to die. As a matter of fact, it seemed a welcome solution."

It was about this time, that I chanced to call J.'s pastor in Roanoke—J. had been on my mind ever since our conversation in the parking lot—and I heard of her wretched status. I phoned to invite her to Mount Rogers.

"J., I can't make any promises, but I think we may be able to help. How soon can you get here?"

"Do you have any idea how sick I am?" she asked. "Don't you know I haven't got any money?"

"Don't worry about that now," I said. "Just come."

And so J. did come, and started chelation therapy in April 1979. Eighteen months later she took leave of us in Trout Dale, a happy and much healthier woman and the most miraculously recovered patient who ever came under my care.

What did I do for J.? What did I do *to* her? First of all, I accepted the risk of trying chelation therapy on J., who was nearly moribund during the first six weeks at our clinic. But many chelation patients come to us in close-to-death condition: "You're my last hope," we hear over and over again. In those cases, where all other treatments have failed, the patients and I often share a "nothing to lose" attitude.

No doctor likes to initiate treatment *after* the patient is so seriously ill that he or she hovers at death's door. But we try.

J. came to us late because, like so many others, she had never heard of the chelation alternative until it was (almost) too late.

For weeks she showed no signs of improvement with chelation. Finally, the treatments began to take hold. Her progress was slow but steady thereafter, and always inspirational.

"No one here is as sick as I was," she would greet other arriving patients, "and look at me now. I'm alive."

To this day, J. is a local legend around the Mount Rogers Clinic. She remains our most striking example of what can be achieved with chelation once blood circulation is restored in blocked arteries.

A prominent cardiovascular surgeon on the teaching faculty of a nearby medical school examined J. in Winston Salem, North Carolina, when she was about to leave us.

"This lady has a remarkable story," wrote the doctor. "She has completely healed necrotic places on her feet, which were obviously caused by her atherosclerosis."

This physician called me to say, "There is nothing I could have done any better, even with vascular surgery. Most patients with her severity of disease would have long since had to have their legs amputated."

The dramatic case history and recovery of J., impressive as it is, is but one of tens of thousands of similar striking reports in the medical files of other chelating physicians which detail equally striking recoveries.

With each passing year in the last decade, increasing numbers of trail-blazing physicians (more than 1000 in the United States alone) have begun practicing chelation. The results? No one has done a statistical survey, but I do not personally know of any physician who has used EDTA chelation therapy for any length of time, in the actual treatment of patients with atherosclerotic vascular disease, who is not convinced of both its effectiveness and safety.

But to the continued frustration of doctors like myself, who year after year demonstrate the clinical effectiveness and safety of chelation therapy, this treatment is still ignored—derided, even—by most mainstream physicians. While there is nothing about chelation that smacks of quackery (it cannot be administered by anyone other than a fully licensed medical doctor) it is still shunned by the medical establishment. Why?

An inherent conservatism within the medical profession often serves to protect the public from ineffective, fraudulent, and potentially harmful therapies. On the other hand, it also slows the acceptance of new medical advances, sometimes for decades.

In this scientific age, a remedy that makes people "feel better" stands little chance of being accepted as valuable unless large-scale double-blind crossover studies confirm what the clinician has observed firsthand. Medical scientists are conditioned to consider anecdotal evidence as unreliable. Testimonials from practicing physicians are treated with disdain. The majority of the medical community, in its smug self-satisfaction, has forgotten that for the most part the laboratory in medicine has followed the kitchen. Many a medical breakthrough was first reported anecdotally. For example, country doctors were feeding their "rundown" patients liver soup long before scientists could identify the cause or cure of pernicious anemia.

In addition, chelation therapy suffers from the "N.I.H." (not invented here) condemnation. Medical advances are supposed to emerge from the richly funded experimental laboratories of the nation's leading medical centers or from grant-rich government-supported research projects, not from the everyday experiences of private physicians.

I believe there is still another and even more important reason chelation therapy is still struggling for recognition. Until very recently, even its staunchest advocates were unable to offer a scientifically defensible explanation for the observed benefits.

While there have been more than 1800 articles in scientific journals about chelation therapy and the usefulness of EDTA, most of these published treatises have concentrated on documenting how well the therapy works, but have given short shrift to the question of how it works. For more than two decades, the dynamics of the treatment have remained a mystery because most reports have focused on its usefulness for lead toxicity, and science had not progressed to the point where the complex biochemistry could be unraveled.

That long-awaited explanation is now at hand. Breakthroughs in an area of medicine known as free radical pathology enable us to provide a coherent, scientific rationale for the many and diverse benefits chelation practitioners have long claimed to have observed.

The free radical concept may be as profound in its implications as the germ theory developed a century ago. Just as the germ theory provided a scientific basis for effective treatment of the major killers of the nineteenth century—the infectious diseases—so the free radical concept provides the groundwork for treatment and prevention of the major killer diseases of this century: atherosclerosis, heart attack, stroke, senility, and cancer. We now know why so many chelated patients report feeling as though their treatments turned back their aging-clocks and restored much of their youthful vigor. For the truth about chelation therapy, as we now understand it, is this: It slows the very aging process itself.

4

Chelation Therapy: What It Is, What It Does, How It Works

Only after the advent of an "acceptable" scientific explanation does an innovative, therapeutic approach stand a chance of being acknowledged by the medical community. Until a physician can explain why a patient has improved with a chosen treatment, his observed cures have little credence among scientists.

A case in point follows. In 1850 Dr. Ignaz Semmelweiss, a Hungarian obstetric physician, reduced maternal mortality rates in his hospital from 25 percent to less than 1 percent simply by requiring attending medical students to wash their hands. Until his death in 1865, Dr. Semmelweiss was plagued by the failure of his colleagues to accept the life-saving benefits of his procedure. It was not until the very year he was buried that an English surgeon, Dr. Joseph Lister, introduced the *principle* of antisepsis to surgical procedures, drawing upon Semmelweiss's observations and the work of Louis Pasteur, who proved that fermenting organisms permeated ordinary air. By the time of Lister's death in 1912, hand washing and antiseptic surgery were commonly accepted practices. But it had taken 50 years.

The perfectly valid recommendations of these two physicians might have been ignored even longer if Pasteur's explanation—the germ theory—had not been accepted by the medical community. Now even school children know about germs and understand that cuts, scrapes, and bruises must be kept clean.

In the 100 years since Pasteur made medical history, there has not been so profound a discovery until the recent development of the concept of *free radical pathology* as the underlying cause of the major degenerative diseases associated with aging.

The free radical concept of aging, first postulated by Dr. Denham Harman in 1962, is this century's major medical advance inasmuch as it provides a cohesive explanation of seemingly contradictory epidemiologic and clinical evidence concerning age-related pathology.

Decades of controversy have pitted scientific theories against each other. One has blamed diet, another the environment, still others point to stressful lifestyles to explain the ever-increasing numbers of Americans being felled by heart attacks, strokes, and cancer. Some have said it's because we are living too long. Still others claim it is because we are living too well—not enough hard work and exercise. Most blame some combination of all the above, plus some as yet little understood factors such as genetic tendencies or over-exposure to carcinogenic chemicals or radiation.

It was not until comparatively recently that researchers had access to the sophisticated technology that enabled them to trace biochemical pathways at the most elemental molecular level to unravel the diet-stress-environment-radiation puzzle.

The dramatic result has been a breakthrough in our understanding of the causes of the major diseases of aging, and a sound scientific basis for the use of nutrition and the modification of stress and lifestyle factors in the treatment and prevention of degenerative ailments. It may even be possible to slow the very aging process itself. The free radical theory of aging introduces a fresh principle: that whether or when one succumbs to a degenerative disease (such as atherosclerosis) depends mainly on the body's ability to defend itself against ongoing free radical attack. While the maximum life-span for a species or an individual appears to be predetermined by genetics (DNA coding), free radicals have a decided influence on whether the limit is reached or not.

We can also posit a sound scientific basis for EDTA chelation therapy. But before we get into that, let us cover some basics—what chelation is and what it does—before how we think it works.

Here are the questions people most often ask when they first learn of chelation, and the answers I give them:

Q: How do you pronounce chelation?

A: With a hard *k* sound: *key-LAY-shun.*

Q: What is chelation therapy?

A: To repeat what was said in the introduction, it is a medical treatment that improves metabolic and circulatory function by removing toxic metals (such as lead and cadmium) and abnormally located nutritional metallic ions (such as copper and iron) from the body. This is accomplished by administering a synthetic amino acid, ethylene-diamine-tetra-acetic acid (EDTA), by an intravenous infusion using a tiny 25-gauge needle.

The verb "chelate" is derived from the Greek noun *chele,* which is the claw of a crab or lobster. Thus "chelation," a natural process, is the pincerlike binding of chelating substances to metallic elements.

Q: Why is chelation a "natural" process?

A: Chelation is a basic life process that enables all growing things and living organisms (including plants) to assimilate and make use of essential inorganic metallic elements. Chelation is nature's marriage ceremony: It weds two substances from totally different chemical worlds—the organic and inorganic—into a compatible working partnership.

Chlorophyll, the plant-greening pigment, is a chelate of magnesium. Hemoglobin, the oxygen-carrying pigment of red blood cells, is a chelate of iron. The chelation process is involved in the formation and function of many enzymes—the protein catalysts that control most of your body's vital biochemical functions.

Industry has made good use of the chelation principle. Chelates are used in household detergents, for example, to reduce the "ring around the bathtub" scum buildup. Chelates binding with magnesium and calcium soften hard water. In much the same way, EDTA pulls abnormal metal ions out of the body, thus reducing the production of free radicals (which will be explained in this chapter) and preventing the conditions under which scum builds up on blood vessel walls. This is an oversimplified explanation of what happens, but will help initiate understanding of the process.

Q: How does the EDTA work?

A: EDTA is a protein-related amino acid molecule with unique and valuable therapeutic properties, one of which is its powerful attraction for loosely bound metals, especially those that speed free radical damage.

Toxic metals, such as lead and cadmium, are double trouble. They inhibit vital enzyme function (disrupting basic metabolic processes) and also greatly increase free radical production. EDTA binds tightly to many abnormally placed metal ions. It forms a chemical bond that facilitates removal of the metal from sites where it might interfere with normal metabolism or enter into an undesirable chemical reaction.

Q: Isn't it dangerous to have essential nutritional metals such as iron, copper, and zinc removed from the body?

A: When they are where they are supposed to be, essential metals are so tightly bound to the sites of normal activity that they are not easily removed. The metallic ions most apt to be removed by EDTA chelation are those that are loose and free-floating. Because this does not hold true all of the time, qualified chelation specialists are careful to provide nutritional supplements to replace essential metals lost.

Q: I've heard chelation described as a "chemical roto-rooter." Is that correct?

A: It is graphic and colorful, but it is scientifically inaccurate. Hoping to make a difficult subject more understandable, a chelation doctor once described chelation as a kind of liquid plumber—a "chemical roto-rooter" that increases blood flow by reaming calcified plaque out of the arteries.

The explanation stuck, and it has haunted chelation specialists ever since. The "chemical plumber" theory is totally invalid, for although EDTA is certainly a calcium chelator, its affinity for calcium is far lower than it is for metals such as iron, copper, lead, cadmium, etc. EDTA will quickly drop calcium to pick up one of these other metals. Furthermore, calcium, as we will see, plays but a minor role in plaque formation.

Q: What does chelation do for the patient?

A: Chelation therapy has been proven to increase blood flow throughout the body. It has been reported to improve liver function, improve blood cholesterol ratios, lower blood fats, reduce blood pressure, reduce leg cramps, improve vision, relieve angina pains, relieve symptoms of senility, heal ulcers caused by poor circulation, forestall heart attacks and strokes, relieve symptoms of arthritis, relieve symptoms of Parkinson's disease and multiple sclerosis, improve memory, and reduce the incidence of cancer.

Q: How much does blood flow increase as a result of chelation?

A: Enough to relieve symptoms, promote healing, and improve the quality of life.

It takes only very slight vascular changes to significantly alter blood flow. Of the thousands of arteries in the body, most are so slender that they have passage space no wider around than a human hair. Most capillaries are so narrow that single blood cells must fold themselves in half to squeeze through. Such diminutive pathways block easily—and small changes may unblock them.

A long-established scientific law states that with perfect laminar flow (fluids moving easily through a thin, smooth conduit) a mere 19 percent increase in the diameter of a vessel will double the flow rate.

But the blood vessels in most of our patients are not thin and smooth: they are usually filled with plaque and, as such, are turbulent conduits. Poiseuille's Law of Hemodynamics tells us that in the presence of turbulence, it takes something less than a ten percent increase in diameter for a doubling of blood flow.

Q: How does chelation increase blood flow?

A: EDTA is similar to aspirin insofar as we simply do not know all the mechanisms involved. Aside from its "buddy-up" action with toxic heavy metals and other abnormal metallic ions, at present we are uncertain of all its beneficial properties.

A recently published article by chelation specialists Dr. Garry Gordon and Dr. Robert Vance, lists more than 20 physiological and biochemical actions of EDTA within the human body, any one of which has the potential to dramatically improve physiological function and/or increase blood flow.

EDTA chelation therapy might, for example, improve arterial elasticity by reducing the number of cross-linkages in the connective and elastic tissues comprising the arterial walls. The artery would then be better able to relax and dilate. Blood flow would increase without existing plaque being affected. Some such cross-linkages are caused by metallic ions bridging large protein and connective molecules. Chelation therapy can also reduce nonmetallic cross-linkages that occur abnormally between large molecules such as sulfhydryl (sulfur to sulfur) cross-linkages.

There is good evidence that EDTA exerts a beneficial effect on the metabolism of individual cells by enhancing cellular use of oxygen and other nutrients, even in the presence of compromised blood flow and diminished oxygen. This effect has been documented experimentally.

Dr. Bruce Halstead, an eminent toxicologist, has reported that EDTA chelation reduces excess free ionic calcium in body tissues, thus slowing its deposition in arterial walls and other diseased tissues.

EDTA restores the normal production of prostacyclin (the "Teflon" of the arteries), which prevents spasms, blocks clots, reduces platelet "stickiness," and improves blood flow, even in diseased arteries. Prostacyclin production turns off in the vicinity of free radical activity.

Which takes us to the most important action of all (not mentioned in the Gordon/Vance article), the fact that EDTA can reduce the localized rate of free radical reactions in blood vessels and elsewhere by removing metallic catalysts of lipid peroxidation.

Peroxidized fats (or lipids, as fats are called scientifically) are rancid—they have combined with oxygen via a free radical catalyzed reaction, releasing mutagenic substances that in their turn oxidize further, creating still more free radicals, and triggering a potentially out-of-control chain reaction.

To grasp the significance of the free radical concept, especially as it pertains to chelation with EDTA, some background understanding of basic biology is helpful. Your body is composed of about 60 trillion cells, each enclosed within an encircling cell wall or membrane.

Cells vary greatly in structure, as well as in function. Those in certain bodily structures—such as the skin, the linings of the intestinal tract, and the blood cells—are continuously worn out and have the ability to replace themselves. Other tissues, such as the brain, nerves, and muscles (including the heart) are made up of nondividing cells that, once worn out, cannot renew themselves. Over time, nonrenewable cells become increasingly damaged in the course of their activities: they age, they die, and they clog tissues and organs and biochemical pathways as cellular "rubbish."

When your cells are damaged, *you* are damaged. When your cells perform inefficiently, *you* perform inefficiently. When enough cells die, *you* die. How do cells get sick and die? They succumb to free radical attack.

A free radical is an oxygen molecule with an odd number of

electrons in the outer orbital ring of one of its atoms. Molecules (and atoms) normally contain an even number of paired electrons. Free radicals differ from all other molecules, ions, and molecular complexes in having an unpaired electron in their structure, a distinction that may seem trivial but that has enormous significance.

If one of the electrons in a pair becomes separated, an imbalance is created. That imbalance makes the resulting molecule (or atom) promiscuously unstable, violently reactive, and very destructive, ready to aggressively attack any nearby substance, setting off further free radical reactions with explosive cell-destroying power. What the free radicals actually do is combine with and react chemically with other molecules that were never meant to be interfered with. Just as outside of us oxygen produces rust on metal surfaces, so, inside of us, unbalanced oxygen molecules "rust" the body.

Free radicals are continuously generated as a result of many essential chemical reactions that occur naturally in the body. These reactions are necessary for life as part of the normal metabolic process. They are a byproduct of the normal use of oxygen, needed to burn fuel (food) and generate energy, and are produced in large numbers in the mitrochondria, the cell's complex "oxygen reactor" or power plant. Free radicals are also generated in the endoplasmic reticulum (detoxification compartment) of liver cells, in white blood cells, and in other locations.

At the same time that oxygen and food are processed in the mitochondria to generate the cell's energy requirements, a flux of free radicals is released. These raiders head for the nearest target—the fatty acids within the mitochondrial membranes—converting them into dangerous peroxidized fats which, in turn, produce even more free radicals.

Uncontrolled, these free radicals can wreak havoc. They are deadly marauders that damage cells by breaking down delicate cell walls, by damaging important protein enzymes, and by ravaging the sensitive structures of the mitochondria so that it is no longer an efficient energy producer. Free radicals have a lifespan of microseconds and their concentration in any site at any moment is minuscule, but they will attack anything in their vicinity with amazing speed.

To appreciate how deadly free radicals are, consider this: Should you be exposed to excessive radiation, you would be made sick by the free radicals produced in your vital tissues by the high-energy radiation. Any time your body is exposed to nuclear radiation—or excessive x-rays—it is free radical damage you must fear.

There is absolutely no way to escape ongoing exposure. Even before the nuclear age, man was constantly subjected to radiation. One quart of ordinary ozone on a sunny day contains about 1 billion free radicals of a highly dangerous type. Cosmic radiation from the sun and stars continually filters through the atmosphere, subjecting our bodies to low-intensity free radical exposure.

Contrary to what most people believe, it is not this external radiation that is most worrisome. Anti-nuke pickets at the Three Mile Island nuclear reactor site might have been surprised to learn that even those persons living closest to the plant were damaged more by their own normally produced internal free radicals than by those from escaping radiation. We are all subjected to continuous internal radiation from highly reactive free radical molecules that are regularly produced within human cells in the normal course of daily life, as a consequence of eating and breathing. How then, does man survive?

As you might suspect, nature has provided us with exquisitely designed survival equipment. Every cell that deals with oxygen is equipped with an anti-oxidant defense system that can quickly and efficiently scavenge and inactivate most free radicals generated normally in the body.

In a healthy body, free radical reactions are controlled but still allowed to proceed in an orderly fashion as needed for energy production and for detoxification of chemicals, germs, and foreign substances. Several enzymes (including catalase, superoxide dismutase, and glutathione peroxidase in cooperation with other anti-oxidants) keep free radicals from running wild. When functioning properly, these enzymes, in concert with an elaborate system of natural free radical scavengers (including the anti-oxidant vitamins, C and E), dampen free radical chemical reactions, thus allowing the desired biological effect without unwanted cellular or molecular damage.

Without these controls, however, there is unrestrained free radical production. Much like a nuclear chain reaction, when out of control free radicals are generated at an ever increasing rate. When that happens, they disrupt cell membranes, damage essential enzymatic proteins, interfere with transport across cell membranes, and cause mutagenic damage to the genes and chromosomes. All these activities produce very sick—or even malignant—cells.

The damage is cumulative and progressive. If the rate of free radical production proceeds unchecked, eventually the body's natural defenses are overwhelmed. Once the containment threshold is breached, an explosive chain reaction occurs, increasing free radical concentration by a millionfold.

The resulting cell destruction, malignant mutation, and damage to enzymes leads to the whole spectrum of circulatory, malignant, inflammatory, and immunologic disorders that cause the vast majority of age-related illness. The link between free radical activity and malignant change was recognized decades ago, and is currently the basis for much anti-cancer research. The latest work of experimental pathologists suggests the major chronic diseases of Western civilization—including cancer, arthritis, senility, atherosclerosis, and related circulatory disorders—may actually be a form of radiation sickness, the result of continuous internal reactions analagous to those produced by nuclear radiation.

The "China Syndrome" of human pathology results in a "meltdown" of cellular power plants, leading to accelerated aging and premature death. This meltdown can be prevented by adequate anti-oxidant protection from free radicals, much as the control rods in a nuclear reactor keep the rate of energy release from reaching the meltdown stage.

What has all this to do with chelation therapy? EDTA—the substance intravenously injected during chelation treatments—can reduce the production of free radicals by a millionfold. It is not possible for free radical pathology to be catalytically accelerated by metallic ions in the presence of EDTA. Unbound metallic catalysts must be present for uncontrolled free radical proliferation to take place in living tissues. EDTA binds ionic metal catalysts, making them chemically inert and removing them from the body.

Chelation therapy stops excessive free radical production in its tracks, halts the development of free radical disease, and allows the body to repair the damage it has already suffered.

For the individual suffering from atherosclerosis, this means that chelation will curb the abnormal process damaging the arteries, allowing them to heal. Free radicals in blood vessels cause mutation of normal cells to atheroma cells (cells that are benignly tumorous) and promote spasm and clot or thrombosis. Free radicals block production of the hormone prostacyclin, allowing unopposed activity of another hormone, thromboxane, which causes spasm and blood clots in arteries. Red blood cells are trapped in the process. They rupture and release free copper and iron, both potent catalysts of lipid peroxidation that increase the rate of the reaction by a millionfold. This chain reaction can be stopped by EDTA, which sweeps up the unwanted metal catalysts, allowing the atheromatous plaque to heal. (More on free radicals as they pertain to atherosclerosis in chapter 6.)

Q: How long does chelation take?

A: Length of treatment varies, of course, with each patient. Chelation is normally undertaken on an outpatient basis, necessitating repeated visits to the doctor's office or clinic. Each treatment takes from three to four hours, if performed properly. The EDTA solution is infused as a very slow drip into a vein on the arm. Patients sit back comfortably in lounge chairs, free to chat, read, nap, or watch television.

A complete course of chelation treatment usually comprises 30 or more visits, depending upon the condition being treated. In severe cases from 50 to 100 treatments have been given, usually not more frequently than every other day. Frequency of treatment and dosages are tailored to individual kidney function and the patient's ability to safely excrete EDTA in the urine. Kidney functions are closely monitored with each infusion to insure against overload. All known medicines cause harm if given in too high a dose or too rapidly. EDTA is no exception.

"Getting chelated" is quite different from other forms of medical treatment. More about that in chapter 11, "The Chelation Experience."

5

To Be—or Not to Be—Chelated: What Every Heart Patient Should Know

Robert Allen Dyer, of Winston Salem, North Carolina, has taken more than his share of lumps. As a prisoner of war in the Philippines, he survived the Bataan death march plus four years of captivity. Upon his release in 1945, Dyer weighed less than 100 pounds. What was left of him was a mess. The first thing doctors did was a gasterectomy; 80 percent of his stomach was removed.

Over the years Dyer was never really healthy. Minor ailments plagued him constantly. Then, five years ago, he began experiencing chest pains. His doctors counseled all the traditional heart ailment strategies.

"First, they advised I change my diet," Dyer recalls. "Next they prescribed drugs. After that they did an arteriogram—and then, finding my main arteries blocked, they said bypass surgery was the only answer."

"We'll get the very best," his family insisted.

Dyer's brother arranged a surgery appointment for him at the Texas Heart Institute in Houston. His surgeon was to be the illustrious Dr. Denton Cooley.

"Wait a minute," Dyer said. "I want another opinion."

Robert Dyer, associate dean of undergraduate studies at Wake Forest University, is an unusually thoughtful, deliberate man with a lifelong habit of turning to books for information needed to make an informed decision.

"I didn't relish the idea of open-heart surgery," he said. "Who does? But more than that, the operation itself made little sense.

What good is bypassing one small segment of an artery when the rest of the circulatory system is undoubtedly affected as well? Since plaque buildup is the end product of a biochemical process, I wondered whether there was a chemical antidote."

After further research, Dyer heard about chelation therapy. It was at this point that I met Robert Dyer for the first time. He had decided to postpone bypass surgery over the objections of his various doctors.

"If anyone recommends chelation therapy to you," one of them had said, "don't you listen. It's dangerous—very dangerous. It can kill you."

Professor Dyer was amused by that remark. "I couldn't understand how chelation could be more dangerous than bypass surgery," he said. "Of my several friends who've had bypasses, one died on the operating table, one has required repeated surgery, and a third tells me if he had it to do all over, he wouldn't."

Within weeks after starting chelation treatment at the Mount Rogers Clinic, Professor Dyer was convinced he had made the right choice.

"Being stubborn paid off," he said. "I'm breathing easier, walking straighter, feeling no pain, and am mentally sharper than ever."

After observing them closely for many years, I am convinced that chelation patients are not like other patients. They tend to be tough-minded individualists. Like Professor Dyer, most of them are independent and strong-willed, sufficiently self-confident to stick with their convictions despite considerable pressure to conform. (Many of them, like Dyer, opt for chelation against their doctor's advice, not to mention that of well-meaning relatives and friends.)

The past ten years have spawned both a new brand of medicine—holistic—and a new breed of patients—shoppers.

People are more medically sophisticated, and growing numbers now approach the medical marketplace as wary consumers. When a practitioner recommends a treatment, they want to know what they are buying.

Not nearly as reluctant as their parents to challenge doctors, many have discarded the traditional submissive patient stance in favor of dealing with their physicians on a more equal footing. They no longer see the physician as God, and they insist on an active voice in their care and cure. I, for one, welcome this new trend.

As I've previously mentioned, I'm accustomed to facing knowledgeable, well-read men and women. Many come from rural provinces but are not at all provincial. Most patients I see are unusually well-informed about their condition and the alternatives available to them. Nevertheless, I routinely block out close to an hour for all new patients—enough time for a constructive dialogue about their health problems and an objective discussion of their various options.

I assume that my readers are equally inquisitive and equally eager to be given the facts. But even men and women knowledgeable about cardiovascular disease, with better than average comprehension of the circulatory system, seldom know all that is necessary to make an informed treatment decision. Atherosclerosis is not that simple a subject.

If you think you are sufficiently informed, you might save time by skipping this chapter. But before you do, take the following eight-statement test.

No fair guessing. When you've chosen an answer, you should also know *why*. If you get eight out of eight correct, wonderful. You can skim through the chapter. If not, it's required reading.

1: Breathing difficulties, chest pains, or leg cramps are invariably associated with atherosclerosis. True or false?

2. The primary cause of most heart attacks is blocked circulation due to atherosclerotic plaque. True or false?

3: "Hardening" of the arteries is a natural physiological consequence of aging. True or false?

4: Substituting margarine for butter and giving up eggs are effective ways to reduce serum cholesterol levels. True or false?

5: Low cholesterol diets reduce the risk of atherosclerosis. True or false?

6: Vigorous sports and physical activity will protect one from developing atherosclerosis. True or false?

7: Hardening of the arteries begins with the build up of calcified fatty deposits to form plaque. True or false?

8: Chelation removes abnormal deposits of calcium from arterial plaque. True or false?

Ready to discover how well you did?

Every one of the above statements is *false*. Not one is *true*.

If you did not get every one of them right, now is the best time to learn not just how chelation works, but how your body works, too. Do not wait until you are under the pressure of time—wracked with pain or facing surgery—to find out what you need to know.

Let's go back over the test, explaining the why behind the false statements.

1. Breathing difficulties, chest pains, or leg cramps are invariably associated with atherosclerosis.

False. You can have advanced atherosclerosis without these expected symptoms. On the other hand, you can have chest pain and *not* have heart disease. While exertion-related chest pain, leg cramps, or shortness of breath are the most common symptoms of atherosclerosis and coronary artery disease, many conditions other than heart trouble can cause chest pain.

Gallbladder disease, hiatal hernia, and shingles are three ailments in which the pain can be remarkably similar to that of heart disease.

Cardiospasm, resulting from an irritation to part of the esophagus, is sometimes hard to distinguish from true angina.

Chest pain can stem from a mild rib inflammation, or from athritis in the joints between ribs and spine or between ribs and breastbone. There is a condition known as nerve root syndrome (pressure or irritation of a nerve root as it exits from the upper spine, resulting from neck strain or "whiplash" injury) that can cause chest pains or anginalike pains in the arms.

Less usual, but still worth mentioning, are chest pains resulting from unsuspected broken ribs brought on by a bout of coughing. Food poisoning, or sleeping with arms or shoulders in an unnatural position, or excessive air swallowing can also cause chest pains.

Aerophagics (or "air swallowers"), much like people who hyperventilate or have overbreathing habits, are often victims of anxiety and emotional tension. Aerophagia and hyperventilation may produce symptoms similar to those of serious circulatory ailments and depression, nervous upset, or other psychological traumas can intensify symptoms that mimic heart disease.

Then there are the many persons who have experienced unsuspected "silent" heart attacks. Until a cardiogram taken during a routine physical exam uncovers evidence of a past coronary event, such individuals often assume they have simply had a bad case of indigestion, or an arm or neck muscle cramp. Sometimes they recollect no symptoms at all.

Typical symptoms of circulatory problems that people frequently do not associate with atherosclerosis are fingers or toes that are often cold, gradual or transient memory loss, and impotence.

No one should decide on his own whether he or some member of his family has atherosclerosis or a heart problem. But special tests can usually determine the presence of coronary artery disease, or else the real cause of symptoms that cause concern.

So when you become nervous about your cardiac functioning, do not assume that it *is* heart disease or that it is not.

2: The primary cause of most heart attacks is blocked circulation due to atherosclerotic plaque.

False. The degree of arterial blockage has never been completely correlated with either heart attacks or symptoms of coronary artery disease, although mechanical blockage is one important cause.

Heart attacks—or myocardial infarctions—may be triggered by either a mechanical blockage (an embolism, a clot, or plaque) that causes a complete cutoff of the heart muscle's blood supply or by a coronary artery spasm, which also causes sudden blood stoppage or by both events occurring simultaneously. In either event, malfunction results from compromised blood flow and oxygen supply. Heart muscle cells are damaged and often irreversibly infarcted, leading to a scarred, nonfunctioning heart muscle.

Angina pains, sometimes leading to a myocardial infarction, are now considered most often to be the result of spasm superimposed on preexisting partial plaque blockage. Heart attacks, however, have been well documented in the complete absence of plaque, with perfectly normal arterial function.

Conclusive proof that coronary spasm without plaque buildup can lead to coronary thrombosis and myocardial infarction has recently been reported. In the July 28, 1983, issue of the *New England Journal of Medicine*, a report was given of a 29-year-old woman who had a history of anginal-type chest pain. Coronary artery ateriograms were performed and the first injection of dye showed no plaque with a completely normal left coronary artery without any evidence of atherosclerosis or other mechanical obstruction. During a second injection of dye, a few minutes later, a diffuse spasm was seen in the left anterior descending artery. Under direct x-ray visualization, a clot was observed to form in the area of spasm and this patient rapidly developed a full-blown myocardial infarction with muscle death. (The doctors got her heart beating again and the patient lived.) This recent report documents the first occasion during which the entire process from spasm through thrombosis and subsequent heart muscle death took place with physicians watching.

It now appears that in a surprisingly significant number of cases, coronary artery spasm or primary metabolic failure of the myocardium (heart muscle) triggers a heart attack in the complete or relative absence of atherosclerosis. Numerous earlier reports of normal arteriograms in patients with myocardial infarctions support the conclusion that spasm without atherosclerosis is not at all unusual.

Conversely, there have been numerous medical reports of individuals with complete blockage of all three main coronary arteries who had no abnormal heart symptoms at all (an American astronaut, for one example), no angina, and excellent tolerance to strenuous physical exertion. Such cases are found at autopsy following accidental death or death from causes other than cardiovascular disease. When three astronauts perished in the tragic Project Apollo launching-pad fire on January 27, 1967, postmortem examinations revealed all three of these men, supposedly in superb health, showed signs of atherosclerotic disease—one with so advanced a case he would have been a bypass surgery candidate had he ever experienced symptoms.

The free radical shut down of prostacyclin production causes unopposed spasm of blood vessels and an increase in platelet accumulation, leading to clotting. This explains why angina or myocardial infarction frequently occurs after a fatty meal replete with peroxidized fatty acids that cause an explosion of free radical activity. Free radical pathology now appears to be the missing link.

While most people are familiar with dangers to the heart posed by plaque accumulations inside the arterial walls, all too few are aware of the equal or greater danger from arterial spasm. More to the point, there is a general lack of public awareness as to what causes arterial spasm and the preventive measures that might ward it off.

Improper calcium/magnesium ratios within the arterial muscle cells appear to be one important causal factor leading to arterial spasm. The heart muscle is also unable to pump rhythmically and adequately when intracellular magnesium is low and calcium is high.

A proper ratio of calcium outside cells to magnesium inside cells must exist in order for proper contraction and relaxation of muscle cells to occur. This is true for both the heart pumping muscles and for the muscle fibers that encircle the arteries and control blood flow.

Calcium (and sodium) is in higher concentration outside muscle cells and magnesium (and potassium) is more concentrated within cells when the muscle is at rest; for contraction of the muscle fibers to occur, there must be a partial reversal of the calcium and magnesium ratios with calcium entering the cells and magnesium leaving the cells. (Sodium tends to parallel the movement of calcium and potassium moves in concert with magnesium.) To complete the contraction-relaxation cycle, the prior concentration gradients must be restored: this requires a pumping action energized by oxygen. If circulation is compromised, and oxygen supply is reduced, calcium and sodium pumping is slowed, resulting in impaired relaxation and spasm.

The vital question then is: How does the calcium/magnesium ratio get out of whack?

Best evidence is that it occurs partially as a result of the general nutritional imbalances of the typical Western diet. (More about this important topic later.) Ongoing free radical damage also causes calcium to leak through cell membranes.

3: "Hardening" of the arteries is a natural physiological consequence of aging.

False. Many people have the mistaken idea that as one gets older, one's arteries "harden," as though after a limited number of years, the artery's inherent destiny is to become rigid, blocked, and inflexible.

Not so. Hardening of the arteries, while most prevalent in the elderly, is the result of biochemical changes that may actually start early in life. Free radical damage leading to the formation of atheromas (benign arterial tumors) and leading to cross-linkage and calcium deposition can be attributed to the high fat, highly refined (white flour, white sugar, white rice) diet of industrialized nations.

4: Substituting margarine for butter and giving up eggs are effective ways of reducing cholesterol levels.

False. Margarine and egg substitute manufacturers have successfully popularized a massive public misconception: that a low cholesterol diet lowers blood cholesterol because of a decreased consumption of cholesterol, when it's actually the reduction in harmful fats that turns the trick.

Cholesterol is necessary for many vital functions such as the emulsification, digestion, and absorption of fats, the synthesis of sex hormones, the production of Vitamin D via an interaction with sunlight, and the protection of part of the lipid membrane surrounding every cell. Cholesterol not only enters the body as food, but is also manufactured by the liver and other organs.

Two-thirds of all the body's cholesterol is normally produced by the body's own cells and does not come from dietary cholesterol intake. Recent research shows that much of the cholesterol in deposits of atherosclerotic plaque is produced within the body and is not derived from food cholesterol directly. Some is produced within the plaque itself.

5: Low cholesterol diets reduce the risk of atherosclerosis.

False. Controlled clinical trials have failed to prove a connection between the consumption of saturated fats and high cholesterol foods with the development of atherosclerosis or heart disease. In fact, a six-year study released in 1978, the Multiple Risk Factor Intervention Trial (MRFIT), costing nearly $115 million in research funds, has made it clear that the battle against coronary heart disease cannot be won merely by cutting down on dietary cholesterol and saturated fat.

In the MRFIT study, approximately 12,000 men at risk for coronary death were randomly assigned to two groups: those in the SI (specific intervention) group were encouraged to adhere to diets designed to lower serum cholesterol levels. Anti-hypertensive medications were prescribed as indicated. Those in the UC (usual care) group received usual medical treatment, but were given no specific dietary intervention or advice to modify other risk factors.

After six years, the men in the SI group achieved a lower serum cholesterol and blood pressure, but with no improvement in death rate. Total death rates and coronary heart disease (CHD) mortality were nearly identical in the two groups, results which dealt a fatal blow to popular hypotheses claiming heart disease is caused primarily by eating too much meat, eggs, butter, whole milk, and other foods containing cholesterol.

More recently, the *American Journal of Clinical Nutrition*, after a comparison of the rate of heart disease and food habits in thousands of people, announced no link could be found between dietary cholesterol and heart trouble.

In fact, several studies have shown that traditional methods for lowering serum cholesterol via diet or using drugs are at best worthless, and at worst, dangerous. One drug commonly used for this purpose was found to increase death rates.

Such findings are in line with current observations that cholesterol is an excellent, fat-soluble, anti-oxidant, free radical scavenger, produced in the body to control undesirable free radicals. Total body cholesterol, as reflected by blood levels of cholesterol, is determined not by dietary cholesterol, but by cholesterol production in the body as a protective response to destructive free radical damage.

Undesirably high serum cholesterol levels, therefore, are not the *cause* of a problem, but the *result* of a problem—an indication of ongoing free radical damage, and for that reason closely related with atherosclerosis.

6: Participation in vigorous sports and strenuous physical activity provides protection against the development of atherosclerosis.

False. Autopsies performed on highly active people, such as marathon runners, have disclosed far advanced atherosclerosis with extensive arterial plaque buildup, although these people rarely exhibited symptoms of disease. Similar investigations of highly mobile populations, such as the nomadic members of the Masai tribes in Africa who routinely walk between 20 and 30 miles a day, have also uncovered a surprisingly high incidence of atherosclerosis in a people long thought to be free of this disease. The Masai diet is high in peroxidized fat and oxidized cholesterol.

That is not to suggest that regular exercise is without benefit, or that devotion to an exercise program is a waste of time. The physically active lifestyle of the Masai is a good example of the protective effect of exercise. Like other super-active people, the Masai, while not immune to plaque buildup, rarely suffer symptoms of arterial blockage from this condition.

It seems that physical exercise has a protective effect, preventing arterial occlusion by promoting collateral circulation around the blocked arteries, or by causing compensatory expansion of the plaque-clogged arteries. While exercise has not been proven to stop plaque buildup, it does improve the ratio of HDL (high density lipoproteins) cholesterol to total cholesterol, meaning HDL percentage (the "good" guy portion) increases in relation to total cholesterol. This is thought to have some retarding effect on disease development.

Individuals who maintain high levels of physical activity have many fewer symptoms of atherosclerosis, and fewer atherosclerotic-related deaths, even when they in fact have extensive arterial plaque.

Indeed, other newly published research also suggests that vigorous exercise reduces the risk of sudden death from coronary heart disease. When a research team at the University of Washington in Seattle and the University of North Carolina in Chapel Hill evaluated activity levels among 1250 persons who died suddenly and unexpectedly of heart disease in 1980, they found sudden death victims had participated less in high-intensity leisure time exercise—jogging, chopping wood, swimming in a pool, singles tennis or squash—than a matched group, who were more active and had a lower sudden death incidence.

In another study, it was found that bus drivers who sat all day had a much higher heart attack rate than did bus conductors who were on their feet all day, running up and down steps on double-decker buses. Furthermore, when Dr. Ruth K. Peters of the University of California studied 2779 Los Angeles policemen and firemen, she found the incidence of heart attack can be dramatically lowered with 20 to 30 minutes of vigorous exercise three or four times a week. It seems that exercise does help to protect one from the harmful effects of atherosclerosis, but it does not prevent the disease from developing and laying the groundwork for the harm it will eventually cause—perhaps in the case of the physically active person in old age rather than middle age.

7: Hardening of the arteries begins with the build-up of calcified fatty deposits called plaque along the inside wall of coronary arteries.

False. The initial event in arterial disease is damage to the arterial lining, resulting from blood flow stress, routine wear and tear, or free radical damage. To understand the basic concepts underlying the development of atherosclerosis, visualize these cells within the arterial walls abnormally multiplying until they form a benign tumor, a growth akin to the cellular proliferation seen in cancer. These arterial wall cells mutate in response to free radical damage to the genes contained in the nucleus, identical to the way in which atomic radiation causes mutations. An occasional cell loses its ability to control cell division and multiplication, resulting in uncontrolled, tumorlike growth.

The tumor (atheroma) thus formed is nonmalignant, and will not metastasize or spread to other parts of the body. But it is nonetheless an unwelcome, space-occupying mass on the inside of the artery, which accumulates collagen, elastin, and other connective tissue constitutents.

When this growth exceeds its blood supply of oxygen and nutrients, it begins to break down in the center, becoming decayed or necrotic, and gradually gathers deposits of cholesterol and calcium. As it grows into what we call plaque, it becomes progressively firmer and more rigid. Calcification is actually a late occurrence in plaque formation—not the initial event.

8: Chelation removes abnormal deposits of calcium from arterial plaque.

False. Before the free radical cause of degenerative disease was known, it was tempting to hypothesize that EDTA chelation had its major effect on calcium metabolism. We now know that calcium is just another link in the chain of cause and effect created by free radical damage.

EDTA can influence calcium in many ways, but the calcium-chelation connection has been blown out of proportion and has been the major weak link in past explanations of how and why EDTA is a beneficial treatment.

One of the primary reasons, I believe, why chelation has never been accepted by the medical profession at large is the reliance of most chelation advocates—lacking any other justification for observed improvement in patients—on unsubstantiated "roto-rooter" types of explanations, which have merely destroyed credibility with knowledgeable scientists.

Newly emerging scientific discoveries now enable us to demythologize the calcium-chelation connection, so we shall devote the next chapter to a more thorough investigation of this entire issue.

6

The Calcium-Chelation Misconception

Let us clear up a major—and most damaging—misconception about chelation therapy. It does not strip calcium out of plaque or calcified "hardened" arteries.

In the early days, chelation therapy pioneers, eager to explain the treatment in terms patients could grasp, described EDTA's action as "pulling rivets out of a bridge," or "decementing the lining of blood vessels." These were crude but vivid ways of describing what they thought was happening—that calcium was being dislodged and drained from "hardened" and plaque-clogged arteries.

Ever since, doctors have stressed the removal of calcium as the underlying reason for chelation "payoffs." This is both scientifically inaccurate and, to a large degree, responsible for delaying universal acceptance of chelation therapy.

Why then have doctors stuck with the calcium-chelation connection when it is highly hypothetical and nebulous, and vulnerable to the justifiable criticism of knowledgeable biochemists and cardiaovascular physiologists?

The use of chelation therapy with EDTA for atherosclerosis was not discovered or developed in a research lab, a teaching hospital, or a university medical school. It evolved in doctors' offices—a suspect setting in the view of the majority of physicians who have far more respect for new modalities that emerge from academia.

Most physicians in private clinical practice were trained many years ago, prior to the introduction of intensive biochemistry in medical schools. They are far more interested in helping patients regain health than in delving into the complex biochemistry responsible for therapeutic effects. The notion that calcium removal shrinks plaque was a convenient explanation that fit best with what was known at the time.

Until recently, most published scientific references to EDTA, relating to either industrial or medical applications, concerned its effect on calcium. EDTA's ability to abstract calcium has freed consumers from "ring around the bathtub" and "ring around the collar"; cardiologists and internists value it in that regard, knowing it to be useful for lowering calcium in patients with life-threatening high blood calcium. The FDA-approved package insert specifies EDTA's use as a calcium chelator for hypercalcemia, caused by advanced metastasized bone-dissolving cancers, and digitalis toxicity (potentiated by calcium).

Degenerative diseases have long been linked to calcium-related excesses. It is well established that as people age, they accumulate calcium deposits in unwanted places, especially in arteries and arterial plaque. EDTA's proven calcium-lowering ability, coupled with demonstrable improvement in the condition of patients so treated, led to the seemingly reasonable conclusion that "zapping" calcium out of the hardened areas was the way EDTA worked.

With 20/20 hindsight, it is easy to ridicule so simplistic a notion. Although EDTA is certainly a calcium chelator, its affinity for calcium is far less than for many other metals such as iron, copper, lead, mercury, cadmium, and aluminum. EDTA will quickly drop calcium to pick up one of these other metals, and will transport it out of the body through the kidneys. Serious investigators, noting that the amount of calcium removed by one infusion of EDTA is less than half a gram—not much more than would normally be excreted by the body in that one day—remained rightly skeptical.

The explanation satisfied the uninitiated, made chelation appear flaky to the sophisticated, and discredited not only the proponents of the calcium-chelation connection concept, but the therapy as well. Thus the baby was thrown out with the bath water. Not believing the tale of how it worked, most well-trained professionals chose to dismiss tales of how well it worked as equally fanciful.

After more than 20 years, the most expedient route to bringing chelation into the mainstream of medicine might be to bury it along with its tortuous history, and begin afresh, to "rediscover" and rename the entire process in light of current new knowledge. I have no doubt, were this to happen, that chelation therapy would, under its new name, be hailed overnight as the medical breakthrough the world has been waiting for.

Since that does not seem feasible, our best alternative is to replace misconceptions with an accurate, scientifically supportable, updated rendition of what EDTA does and does not do. There *is* a calcium-chelation connection, but it is of secondary importance compared with EDTA's impact on free radicals. It is the free radical-chelation connection that is most responsible for improvement in individuals with disordered calcium metabolism, atherosclerosis, and all degenerative diseases.

If EDTA does not simply "pull out calcium rivets" or "decalcify" plaque, how then does it reverse symptoms of atherosclerotic disease?

To summarize what is currently known about the cause and effect relationships in atherosclerosis: The initiating event in hardening of the arteries is a localized injury to the lining of a blood vessel wall. This superficial loss of cells occurs repeatedly during normal daily activities from the following three causes:

- (1) Ongoing "injuries" of a low magnitude are a normal result of the stress of blood flow and routine wear and tear. Such localized injuries are more frequent and severe in the presence of high blood pressure. Healthy defenses rapidly heal these small defects.
- (2) Free radicals cause damage to blood vessel walls. Atherosclerosis is speeded by the presence of free radicals, which have the ability to proliferate, producing a cascade of other free radicals—a case of a poison producing more poison.
- (3) Ongoing blood vessel injury may also be immunologic. That is, the body's immune system, which is essential for proper resistance to disease-causing organisms and environmental contaminants, may inappropriately attack healthy cells.

For a variety of reasons, also related to excessive free radicals, a blood vessel injury can result in a tumorlike atheroma rather than normal healing. The plaque, which has no blood vessels within, continues to grow until it becomes so large that adequate oxygen and nutrients cannot diffuse into its core from the surrounding blood. The center of the plaque then degenerates, eventually picking up deposits of calcium and cholesterol. Calcification is a relatively late event in the development of both arteriosclerosis—hardening of the arteries—and atherosclerosis—hardening of the growth or plaque.

While there are quite a number of nutritional and lifestyle factors that contribute to the formation of atherosclerotic plaque and its calcification, we shall deal here specifically with the form of disordered calcium metabolism most directly corrected by EDTA.

Long before abnormal calcium deposits become solidified and visible on x-rays or to the naked eye at autopsy, there is a progressive fine mist of calcium building within cells and connective tissues. The absolute amount of calcium within the body is not the most important factor. Abnormalities first occur in relationships between calcium concentrations such as bone versus soft tissue and in the ratio of calcium to magnesium.

An optimal calcium to magnesium ratio results in a much higher concentration of calcium outside the cells than within. Healthy cells, with active energetic metabolism, are able to maintain an efficient pumping system within their lipid membrane walls that keeps calcium out and magnesium in.

With aging, this concentration gradient deteriorates. Calcium levels increase within the cells as magnesium levels decrease, partly because of the gradual breakdown of the cell's pumping mechanism, which can be damaged by many things, including free radicals. Also, free radical damage to the cell wall creates "leaks" that allow calcium to seep in and magnesium to seep out. A healthy cell wall is quite impermeable to these metal ions.

The more calcium leaks into a cell, the more poisoned its metabolism becomes, and eventually crystalline deposits form inside the cell, causing it to die. The more cells that die, the fewer are left to keep the basic life processes going.

Excess intracellular calcium and abnormally high calcium-magnesium ratios speed cell death, especially when blood flow and oxygen delivery become compromised by atherosclerosis. Arterial spasm becomes much more intense and calcium leakage into cells proceeds much more rapidly once the cellular calcium-magnesium ratio is disrupted.

A vicious cycle is set in motion as diminished blood flow and reduced oxygen speed calcium leakage into cells. Intracellular calcium causes muscle cells surrounding arteries to go into more intense spasm, causing further reduction in blood flow and oxygenation, speeding calcium influx, and on and on.

This self-perpetuating process underlies the success of recently introduced calcium "blockers," such as nifedipine and verapamil, which slow the entry of calcium into muscle cells. The calcium "blockers" work by an entirely different mechanism than EDTA and they have no effect on calcium removal nor on free radical damage.

In addition, impairment of the calcium-magnesium pump allows more ionized calcium to enter the cell, activating an enzyme that leads to the production of prostaglandin-related leukotrienes, a chemical reaction that releases free radicals. Leukotrienes are potent inflammatory substances that attract white blood cells to the area which produce free radicals as bullets to attack foreign invaders. When excessively stimulated by leukotrienes, white blood cells run amok and initiate excess free radical production, which causes increasing inflammatory damage to healthy tissues. Small blood vessels dilate, causing swelling, edema, and leakage of red blood cells and platelets through blood vessel walls, which result in microthrombi (microscopic clots). Some red blood cells then hemolyze, releasing free copper and iron, which in turn catalyze an increase of free radical destruction to lipid membranes in the vicinity by a millionfold, triggering another vicious cycle.

The accumulation of intracellular and connective tissue calcium is further speeded by the Vitamin D activity of certain cholesterol oxidation products created by free radical reactions. This Vitamin D-like activity produces a form of localized Vitamin D toxicity in cells and tissues, the effect of which is to speed calcium deposits.

Once free radical production exceeds the body's threshold to protect itself, metabolic breakdown, cellular damage, and tissue calcification all take place more rapidly, even exponentially. It now appears that calcium deposition is just another link in the chain of cause and effect created by free radical damage. EDTA can influence and speed removal of calcium deposits in many ways as part of the healing process, but not as directly as formerly hypothesized.

EDTA does reduce blood calcium levels during infusion and hastens excretion, but if you look at the 1500 grams of total calcium in the body, the one-third gram excreted is so relatively small—far less than dietary calcium intake on an average day, and barely more than normal daily urinary excretion—that this cannot be the main benefit of the therapy.

During the short time that EDTA is circulating in the body (it has a half life of only one hour), it temporarily lowers blood calcium. The resulting drop in serum calcium provides a stimulus to the parathryoid gland to step up production of parathormone. This hormone, in turn, signals osteoblasts in bone to increase their production of normal bone calcification, drawing on other calcium sources in the body, some, presumably, from pathological deposits. The pulsed, intermittent parathormone stimulation, produced by each chelation, is known to cause a lasting effect on these osteoblasts, of approximately three-month duration. This is a proven effect of EDTA, and one that makes perfect sense, for it provides a hypothetical explanation for the three-month waiting period for complete benefit to occur following a series of intravenous EDTA chelation therapy infusions.

The so-called "90 day syndrome" (the greatest results are often achieved approximately 90 days after the completion of treatment), a commonly noticed phenomenon by both patients and chelating physicians, may also reflect a more important EDTA effect: reduction of free radical damage allowing gradual healing, which also takes months to become evident.

If, as the newest research indicates, the free radical theory of degenerative disease is correct, then reversing free radical pathology would be the key to the treatment and prevention of such major age-related ailments as atherosclerosis.

EDTA chelation is unique in its ability to control free radical reactions and to restore metabolic health by removing toxic heavy metals.

Specifically, EDTA reduces the rate of pathological free radical chemical reactions by a millionfold, below the level at which the body's defenses can take over, and so provides time for free radical damage to be repaired by natural healing.

Let us consider the physiologic effects of EDTA in relation to free radical pathology:

- EDTA controls free radical damage. Free radicals cause cell destruction by initiating chain reactions of lipid peroxidation, which disrupt fatty membranes within and surrounding cells. Lipid peroxidation requires the presence of abnormally located metal ions such as copper and iron. EDTA removes these metal ions, which accumulate with age, and permits normal healing of peroxidative damage by stopping further peroxidation.

- EDTA removes lead and other poisonous metals, restoring normal enzyme functioning. Excessive concentrations of heavy metals cause enzymatic dysfunctions independent of their action as free radical catalysts, with a concomitant loss of cellular homeostasis and failure of vital cell functioning.
- EDTA enhances the integrity of cell membranes. The ability of cells to produce and store energy depends on healthy membranes surrounding each cellular compartment, including each tiny, interior energy factory, called a mitochondrion. EDTA is known to stabilize mitochondrial membranes and to enhance the efficiency of energy metabolism, independent of any effect on blood flow or oxygen.
- EDTA helps reestablish prostaglandin hormone balance, which in turn prevents arterial spasm, blood clots, plaque formation, and arthritis. Prostaglandins are extremely potent hormones, with a half-life measured in seconds, and must be constantly synthesized. The two most important prostaglandins, in relation to blood vessels and atherosclerosis, are prostacyclin and thromboxane. The first reduces the tendency of platelets to stick and cause blood clots and reverses blood vessel spasms; the second does just the opposite—it causes intense spasm and stimulates platelets to become very sticky, converting blood vessel walls to "fly paper." In fact, a proper balance between the two must be maintained to protect against injury and hemorrhage on the one hand, and to maintain normal circulation on the other. Prostaglandins are produced from fatty acids, and production is put into imbalance by destructive lipid peroxidation. EDTA inhibits such lipid peroxidation by chelating out the catalyzing metallic ions.
- EDTA protects the integrity of blood platelets. Platelets are very small, semicellular corpuscles in the blood stream that quickly adhere to areas of injury and release substances that diminish blood loss by forming clots. In the process of clotting, they change shape, tend to become too "sticky," and attach

themselves too readily to the walls of diseased coronary, cerebral, or other arteries. Platelets also release spasm-producing thromboxane. When platelets come in contact with EDTA, their tendency toward over-coagulation is reduced.

- EDTA sweeps up minute molecules of lead, cadmium, mercury, aluminum, copper, iron, and other metals deposited abnormally through the body. Concentrations of metallic ions that have the ability to catalyze free radical chain reactions are so tiny that even the unmeasurable residue in distilled water may initiate such reactions. The addition of EDTA completely blocks these free radical chain reactions that would otherwise occur, by binding metallic ionic catalysts, making them chemically inert, and removing them from the body.
- EDTA normalizes calcium metabolism by reactivation of the enzymes poisoned by lead and other heavy metals. Most important, EDTA neutralizes free radical activity, which converts cholesterol into substances with Vitamin D activity—activity that causes plaque to accumulate calcium.
- EDTA intermittently lowers serum calcium, allowing gradual reversal of abnormal calcification, by stimulating uptake of calcium in bones.
- EDTA increases tissue flexibility by uncoupling age-related cross-linkages. Cross connections between large protein and other connective tissues molecules cause the increasing rigidity and loss of flexibility so common with aging. Cross linkages to enzyme proteins can interfere with normal biochemical activity.
- EDTA encourages overall metabolic efficiency due to the whole range of factors given above.

The development of atherosclerosis, or any degenerative disease, takes decades, and is almost always the result of not one, but a combination of health-destroying factors. In like manner, reversing the process cannot rely on just one "magic bullet." Impaired health can only be restored by therapies that counteract a spectrum of disease-causing factors.

Underlying every known risk factor contributing to the degenerative diseases—from atherosclerosis to cancer—is excess free radical activity with resulting free radical pathology.

Improper diet causes free radical damage; so does smoking, abuse of alcohol and drugs, insufficient exercise, excessive stress, and lack of adequate vitamins, minerals, and trace elements. The key to restoring health is to reverse the free radical pathology, gradually, by adopting health-promoting lifestyle strategies and, if need be, more directly and quickly by a course of chelation treatments.

With our new understanding of free radical chemical reactions, there is now a sound basis for universal acceptance of EDTA chelation therapy.

7

First, the Good News: Other Chelation Payoffs

Is it really true that chelation improves memory, reduces insulin requirements in diabetics, restores sight, increases sexual potency, lessens the aches and pains of rheumatoid arthritis, smooths away wrinkles, reverses senility associated with Alzheimer's disease, and ups longevity?

For many years, it has been downright embarrassing to me, a Harvard Medical School graduate and president of my county medical society, to be in the position of endorsing a treatment that sometimes makes me sound like an itinerant medicine man drumming up sales for a suspect new cure-all.

While I have never represented chelation to be a treatment for any conditions other than those stemming directly from atherosclerosis it is impossible to ignore the other benefits experienced by chelation patients.

One of the great drawbacks to gaining acceptance for chelation has been its literature, history, and lore, crammed as they are with reports that chelation is successful not only in reversing the symptoms of atherosclerosis, but in improving patients' health status in many other, less predictable, ways.

Case in point: Bessie Black.

When 70-year-old Bessie first came to the clinic, she presented a laundry list of health complaints typical of people her age who suffer from atherosclerotic cardiovascular disease.

"There's so much wrong with me, I don't know where to start," she said.

Bessie's daughter, Flora Driscoll, who had all but carried her feeble mother from the car to the office, filled in the medical details. Bessie's clinical history included two heart attacks, chronic pulmonary disease in the form of bronchial asthma and emphysema, severe osteo-arthritis, heart failure, chest and leg pains, bone softening, cataracts in both eyes, insomnia, and lately, mental confusion characterized by extreme forgetfulness.

"Sometimes, I don't even remember Flora's last name," Bessie cried.

"After Dad died," her daughter related, "Mom was okay for a while, but then she got to the point where she couldn't do for herself. She couldn't remember to take her medicine as directed. Sometimes she'd skip it, other times she'd double-up and overdose. She had difficulty expressing herself. She was terribly depressed, and she talked about dizzy spells. If she walked upstairs she'd get terrible pains. Some days she forgot to eat, and we were always afraid she'd walk off and forget how to get home.

"We've had Mom everywhere, but it seems that all the medications and drugs have just added to her problems. Each time they prescribe something that helps one condition, it brings on another.

"Every doctor I've seen has told me Mom will never be able to look after herself or live alone anymore. The last one said it would all be downhill, and that eventually she'd require nursing home care. Do you want to know what he told me? He said, 'Don't look so glum. By that time, she won't know the difference.'"

Many doctors do not like to treat old people. It's frustrating because you can't "cure" old age. But Flora wasn't ready to give up on her mother. When her neighbor, a nurse, told her about chelation, she hoped for a reprieve.

We started Bessie Black's chelation therapy the second week of September, 1981. Ten weeks and 20 treatments later she resumed housekeeping, able to care for herself once more. Better still, Bessie celebrated Thanksgiving by cooking dinner—turkey and all the trimmings—for a houseful of relatives. There was a family reunion that Bessie's kinfolk, 20 in number, are still talking about.

"Some of my folks hadn't seen me in a while, and they couldn't imagine me this much improved," Bessie chuckled.

"I just never get tired of hearing them marvel at how well I look."

Ormal Dettor, 82 years of age, was losing her sight. Remarkably healthy for a woman her age, she was bitter at having to curtail her activities and depressed at the prospect of becoming totally blind.

"I love to read, do needlework, paint, watch TV, visit people. I like to walk, garden, and keep busy," she told me.

"Now, the doctors have told me I have to learn to live like a blind lady. I'll try anything—diet, vitamins, chelation, you name it—that will help me retain some degree of sight."

Mrs. Dettor's medical records confirmed severe macular degeneration, involving problems with central vision in each eye due to atherosclerotic changes in retinal blood vessels on the back surface of the eye. By the time we began chelation treatments, almost all vision was gone from her right eye. Her ophthalmologist had known of other patients suffering with similar macular degeneration who had been dramatically helped by chelation therapy, and so referred Mrs. Dettor to me.

"I just held my breath the first few treatments. I couldn't see a thing out of my right eye, and the other was getting worse. Then, after my fifth treatment, I was at home lying on the sofa. For some reason I raised myself up, closed my left eye, and looked out toward the front door and caught sight of the sky and a neighbor's terrier crossing the lawn.

"I couldn't believe it! I was seeing and with my bad eye. I jumped up and ran outdoors, holding my breath for fear it wasn't true. But when I looked all around, and saw the trees and everything okay, I started yelling 'I can see! I can see!' Let me tell you, I stirred up the neighborhood that day."

It wasn't long before Mrs. Dettor was sewing a bit, and reading again. She can even find names in the telephone directory now. The last time she visited me for a follow-up chelation she had just returned from a trip to India and showed off pictures of herself riding on an elephant.

Without exception, chelation physicians have noted that patients almost invariably enjoy multiple benefits. Most experience symptom relief not only from the one specific ailment for which treatment was undertaken, but also from other, secondary complaints—a lessening of aches and pains, a reduction of joint stiffness, dizziness, ringing in the ears, mental sluggishness, and general fatigue.

Occasionally, there are dramatic results, such as a recovery from acute paralysis, reversal of blindness, a restoration of hearing. Rex Smith of Hinton, Virginia, could not use the telephone without an amplifier prior to chelation; now he can. Bill Dewhirst, who received 35 chelations following a severe heart attack, was astonished to find his gray hair, especially on his chest, gradually turned dark once again. Bill's cardiac ejection fraction, measured by noninvasive isotope rated blood flow test, more than doubled following chelation.

One 67-year-old patient (the only one who requested his name not be used) told me he was able to resume normal sexual function after many years of difficulty. He had been a victim of Peyronie's disease, which is characterized by the formation of hardened scar tissue on one side of the penis causing an erection to be bent an at angle, and making intercourse painful or impossible. After 35 chelations, the scar tissue apparently dissolved completely, and a normal erection was again possible.

At first exposure, many of these recoveries appear miraculous, but to chelation specialists, who have witnessed scores of "can you top this?" case histories, they have become routine. The scientific literature also contains many case histories that document that chelation frequently pays off in unexpected ways.

As early as 1963, *Medical World News* reported that diabetics had reduced insulin requirements after chelation, and monthly or bimonthly infusions of EDTA helped keep complications of their disease under control. According to this medical periodical, Philadelphia heart specialists Dr. Lawrence E. Meltzer and Dr. J. Frederick Kitchell were "excited to discover" that chelation with EDTA offered very positive benefits for diabetics, some of whom were able to discontinue insulin injections for long periods. (In my experience, insulin requirements are usually reduced by approximately half after chelation.)

In addition, the doctor's reported, some diabetics suffering from severe peripheral vascular problems who had developed lower extremity gangrene, were saved from undergoing leg amputations. One such patient, Dr. Kitchell recalled, "ended up walking the entire seven miles of the Atlantic City boardwalk, and couldn't walk a block before we started therapy."

While the physicians were uncertain as to the specific ways in which chelation reversed the course of the disease process, they speculated it had something to do with EDTA's ability to alter the enzyme activity that controls blood sugar formation by segregating and removing toxic metals and by restoring a balance to the essential minerals and trace elements. Iron, zinc, copper, cobalt, and manganese were five metals named as possibly contributing to the pathology of enzyme systems. (We now know that iron and copper are potent free radical catalysts.)

When their studies showed that diabetic patients characteristically have abnormal metal excretion patterns in the urine during chelation—excreting more zinc and less tin than normal patients—this finding added credibility to their speculation. Zinc is involved in the proper functioning of many separate enzyme systems, and it functions as part of the storage mechanism of insulin.

Abnormal metal excretion patterns, by the way, have been noted not only in diabetes, but also in rheumatoid arthritis patients, and in individuals with cancer. This supports recent conclusions that trace metal imbalances that interfere with normal enzyme functioning, may in turn lead to increased free radical activity and the development of many serious degenerative ailments.

According to Dr. John Olwin, a cardiovascular surgeon and formerly a clinical professor of surgery at Loyola University Medical School in Chicago, "It seems reasonable to assume that chelation with EDTA, by removing some of the more than 50 contaminating trace metals that have been found to accumulate within the human body, may revitalize enzyme systems damaged by their presence."

Dr. Olwin, whose speculation preceded by many years current knowledge of the way in which trace metals catalyze free radical activity, was impressed by clinical results with chelation, although he admitted he was unable to explain how specific improvements come about. Nevertheless, he could see no reason why the therapy's incomprehensibility should stand in the way of patients enjoying benefits similar to those he had observed. He began using chelation many years ago, first on patients suffering from obliterative atherosclerosis in their legs. Most of them were candidates for summary amputation.

"We saved many of those limbs," Dr. Olwin has noted. "The necrotic areas were limited; they dropped off; the limbs warmed; the nails and hair began to grow."

Olwin extended treatment to patients suffering from a variety of circulatory diseases, and, along with relief from pain, he reported the healing of ischemic ulcers, a decrease in recurrent thrombophlebitis, and improvement in mental processes.

"In the early stages," reported Dr. Olwin, "we noted that people with gangrenous limbs and gangrenous toes, in some instances were not as mentally sharp as they had been. One executive who had lost his job because of this returned to work after he had been treated with EDTA.

"Some patients note an increased nail and hair growth, and say they've been getting haircuts more often than they did before.

"There's been an increase in libido and potency reported by some patients. One man, a once brilliant, 80-year-old lawyer, had had chronic brain syndrome (senility) for many years and then was chelated. About a year later, his wife called one day to ask, 'Is this supposed to increase sexual desire?' When she was told it's been reported to have that effect, she replied, 'Well, James hasn't been interested in sex for 15 years, and last night he tried to make love to me.'"

Until recently most sex therapists agreed that 90 percent of all cases of impotence are primarily psychogenic—a dysfunction of the mind, not the body. Today, most experts believe at least 50 percent of the time impotency stems from a physiological problem. Erectile failure—the most persistent and troublesome male sexual complaint—is often related to atherosclerosis, which may severely restrict the blood supply to the lower limbs and pelvic area.

Danish psychologist Dr. Gorm Wagner, a specialist in human sexuality research for more than a decade, has linked both impotency and frigidity to constricted blood flow, basing his conclusions on studies that used a penis-linked camera to photograph changes in the sex organs during simulated intercourse.

If there is a circulatory component to some forms of Parkinson's disease, as many specialists believe, that would help explain the reported instances in which sufferers of this ailment have improved after chelation therapy. Although no clinical studies have been done to date, oxygen starvation affects the same parts of the brain as the encephalitis virus infection that in later years can lead to Parkinson's disease.

Another possible mechanism by which chelation might be working to reduce symptoms would be the removal of aluminum from body tissues. Autopsies of Parkinson's disease victims have revealed higher concentrations than normal of aluminum in the affected parts of their brains. Aluminum causes cross-linkages in free radical damaged tissues. It is thought by Dr. Harman that free radical damage-induced oxidation of dopamine receptors is the true cause of one form of Parkinson's. Improvements in symptoms of Parkinson's disease following chelation are not as consistent as seen in patients with proven circulatory disorders, but they occur often enough to warrant further research.

What about the aches and pains of rheumatoid arthritis? Why do patients so often report less discomfort after chelation?

Rheumatoid arthritis is actually a collagen (connective tissue) disease, and chelation is known to restore collagen to a healthier state by reducing cross-linkages, not just those caused by metallic ions such as calcium and aluminum, but also those connected with the increased linking of sulfur atoms on adjacent coils of springlike connective-tissue molecules.

Incidentally, the FDA recently approved an oral chelating agent called d-penicillamine for use in cases of rheumatoid arthritis. This drug, now coming into more widespread use, chelates copper, lead, and other trace elements and is similar to EDTA in some of its actions but is far more toxic. D-penicillamine is under active development in both Europe and the United States. There are high hopes that oral chelates may be the wave of the future, but it is too soon to know for sure.

But do we have an explanation for Bessie Black's recovery from "incurable" senility?

Once a relatively rare problem, "senility" has become epidemic. It is estimated that there are currently 1 million senile persons in the United States. Some leading psychiatrists are predicting 4 million Americans will be similarly afflicted by the year 2020.

Not all cases of "senility" are related to vascular disease. True dementia—medically defined as the deterioration of or the loss of intellectual faculties, reasoning power, and memory, and usually characterized by confusion, disorientation, apathy, and some degree of stupor—can also be the result of a virus, as in the rare (and always fatal) disorder called Creutzfeldt-Jakob disease, or in the genetic disorder Huntington's disease, in Parkinson's disease, or in multiple sclerosis. There is also multi-infarct dementia, caused by multiple little strokes caused by ischemia (blockage) of numerous small areas of the brain. These can be caused by "showers" of debris released from ulcerated plaques in the larger arteries of the neck.

More than half of all so-called dementias, however, are caused by Alzheimer's disease, which results in a progressive deterioration of brain function. Alzheimer's disease, which tends to strike its victims in middle age, results in a relentless form of "brain rot" generally considered to be irreversible.

No less an authority than Dr. Neal R. Cutler, chief of the section on brain aging and dementia of the Laboratory of Neurosciences at the National Institute of Aging, has been quoted as considering Alzheimer's disease "incurable."

Alzheimer's disease extracts a tremendous price. Caring for an Alzheimer patient is a nightmare. He or she is typically paranoid, suspicious, delusional, hostile, irritable, and irrational, insisting on performing tasks such as financial transactions, or driving the family car, long after becoming unable to do so.

Eventually, overburdened families admit they are unable to cope. More than half of all admissions to nursing homes are Alzheimer victims, at an average cost of $17,000 a year.

But is Alzheimer's as hopeless as most scientists claim? Is senility an inevitable consequence of our living longer?

Chelation therapists have valid reasons for a more optimistic outlook. Most now believe Alzheimer's is treatable, and in some cases, reversable. Not only is there clinical evidence to support that view, but also scientific support in the new findings linking trace metal accumulations to Alzheimer-type mental deterioration.

One neurological phenomenon of Alzheimer's disease is the finding of tangled fibers disrupting brain cells on microscopic examination of victims' brains. Dr. Daniel P. Perl of the University of Vermont has found abnormal accumulations of aluminum within the affected brain cells of those neurofibrillary tangles.

Going one step further, a team of researchers from the National Institute of Neurological and Communicative Disorders and Stroke (NINCDS), headed by Dr. D. Carleton Gajdusek, found high accumulations of aluminum in the brains of Chamorro natives of Guam who had died of either amyotrophic lateral sclerosis (ALS) or Parkinsonism dementia.

This population has been closely watched because it has been adversely affected by a high incidence of those two chronic disorders, both of which were previously suspected to be transmitted by a slow-acting virus. For several years, Dr. Gajdusek and his colleagues have been studying the implications of the high levels of aluminum found on the island of Guam.

Because of the similarities between the Parkinsonism dementia syndrome and the presenile form of Alzheimer's dementia, other researchers have kept a watchful eye on these studies. In both disorders, there is an excessive accumulation of aluminum-containing neurofibrillary tangles in the brains of victims. The newest findings confirm Dr. Perl's earliest work correlating high concentrations of aluminum in the brain with the development of these tangles.

Furthermore, NINCDS scientists are exploring the possibility that mild hyperparathyroidism caused by dietary imbalances of calcium, magnesium, and phosphorous could contribute to accumulations of toxic concentrations of aluminum, especially in specific areas of the brain.

These are landmark findings because they confirm what holistic physicians have long been claiming: chronic "subclinical" environmental metal toxicity is one of our important health problems. Toxic metals, such as lead, can be shown to depress our immune systems as well as our brain functions. This breakdown of immunity is related to the onset of cancer, and also causes allergies.

Dr. Carl Pfeiffer, director of the Brain Bio Center in Princeton, New Jersey, has also been researching blood aluminum levels and has found a very high correlation between loss of memory and elevations of blood aluminum.

If aluminum is a contributing factor in Alzheimer's, little wonder this disease has grown to epidemic proportions, affecting more and more people at younger and younger ages. Aluminum, the most common element in the earth's crust, has no known function in our body, but we are absorbing more and more of it through our digestive tracts.

While relatively large amounts of aluminum have always been present in food, there is reason to believe we now get a heavier dose than our bodies can comfortably handle.

Our early ancestors ingested a significant amount of aluminum from the rocks and stones that they used to mill grain into flour. But, we have added aluminum to our diets in great quantities. It is not only in all our junk foods, but also in our water supply and in our drugs. It gets into our foods via the use of aluminum pots and pans, the wrapping of acid foods such as tomatoes in aluminum foil, and the storing of foods in aluminum cans.

Aluminum is a common component of many of today's foods. Among them are processed cheeses (aluminum is added as an emulsifying agent), pickles (as a firming agent), baking soda, and cake mixes (as a leavening agent). It is used in the manufacture of antacids, anti-perspirants, buffered aspirin, and vaginal douches.

Subclinical aluminum poisoning appears to be a substantial, if generally undetected, problem. Antacid tablets, for instance, commonly contain 200 mg or more of elemental aluminum, with a recommended dosage of up to 24 tablets daily, only ten of which would put the user more than 100 times over the presumably acceptable 20 mg a day mean. Similarly, buffered aspirin contains 10-52 mg of aluminum per tablet; a 14-tablet-per-day regimen would also result in high aluminum intake. More and more aluminum num is infiltrating into our environment, some in the form of acid rain, which dissolves aluminum from the soil and from cooking utensils.

The body has historically had good defenses against aluminum intoxication by preventing absorption from the digestive tract. There is now evidence that common dietary imbalances of calcium, magnesium, and phosphorous, with increased Vitamin D intake from fortified foods, have resulted in an increase of aluminum absorption from the intestines. Acid rain has resulted in a greater uptake of aluminum by food plants.

When aluminum gets into the bloodstream, it tends to affect the parathyroid gland, causing a further imbalance of calcium-regulating hormones, which in turn further increases the absorption of ingested aluminum. This self-perpetuating cycle results in higher levels of tissue aluminum than have occurred in past generations. Aluminum can cause cross-linkages between collagen and elastic tissue molecules, increasing rigidity or sclerosis of soft tissues, and speeding that aspect of aging.

Is it purely coincidental that we are witnessing a devastating increase in the incidence of all chronic degenerative diseases at the very same time that toxic metal exposure is at higher levels than ever before?

Quite unlikely, especially since chelation—known to remove

unwanted metallic elements out of the body—has proven remarkably effective for the very ailments now suspected to develop as a result of metal poisoning.

When Dr. Richard Casdorph, assistant clinical professor of medicine at the University of California Medical School in Irvine, an internist and cardiovascular specialist, recently investigated the efficacy of EDTA chelation therapy in brain disorders, he documented a measurable increase in cerebral blood flow in all but one of 15 patients. The statistical probability that this could have been due to random chance or a placebo effect is less than one in 10,000.

Using radioisotopes to measure before and after chelation cerebral blood flow, Dr. Casdorph was able to show for the first time that chelation is unquestionably useful in the treatment of senility where impaired cerebral blood flow is a factor.

One of Dr. Casdorph's subjects was a 76-year-old white female, clinically diagnosed with Alzheimer's disease, with CT scan evidence of cerebral atrophy (brain shrinkage). At the onset of therapy, she was confused and in a vegetative state. After 20 infusions of EDTA, there was "marked improvement in the brain blood flow study, as well as significant improvement in her mental functioning," Dr. Casdorph reported.

Another patient, a 72-year-old lady with a long-standing history of documented cerebral atrophy, was having delusions and hallucinations and at times would not recognize her husband of 50 years. On more than one occasion, after walking out to the sidewalk in front of her home, she had not been able to find her way back into the house. When Dr. Casdorph included her in his study, her husband was considering institutionalizing her.

"After the first six infusions (of EDTA chelation therapy), all of the above mentioned symptoms cleared, the patient was completely oriented and rational," Dr. Casdorph writes. "It was no longer necessary to consider institutionalization. There also occurred some improvement in her vision."

In Dr. Casdorph's view, when toxic metals have accumulated over the years, they impair enzyme reactions and block metabolic pathways, and thus may accelerate the development of age-related degenerative diseases. Chelation, which successfully removes trace amounts of lead, cadmium, and aluminum, may serve to improve cell function.

Canadian investigators have also now found aluminum at above normal levels in the brains of some Alzheimer's victims, and they speculate that senile dementia might more properly be called aluminum dementia. Clinching the metal poisoning tie to Alzheimer's is recent evidence from the University of Toronto that chelating metals from the body either halts or reverses mental deterioration in SDAT (senile dementia of the Alzheimer's type) patients.

When Dr. Donald McLaughlan, professor of physiology and medicine of the University of Toronto, attempted a small clinical trial with an iron chelating agent (deferoxamine), six treated SDAT patients improved, while 11 untreated controls did not, as judged by the Wechsler Intelligence and Memory Scale, signal detection tasks, and an EEG (electroencephalograph). Deferoxamine is most potent as an iron chelator (iron is a free radical catalyst known to accumulate with age) and binds only weakly to aluminum and other metals that speed free radical pathology. If Dr. McLaughlan had used EDTA, I suspect his results would have been even better, since brain cells are highly sensitive to free radical damage.

At Ohio State University, investigators have taken a different approach. They have embarked on a five-year study of Alzheimer's patients to determine the long-term effects of low-aluminum diets in conjunction with agents that limit aluminum absorption.

Incidentally, Dr. Johan Bjorksten, a prominent gerontological researcher, points out aluminum is building up not just in our brains, but in all our tissues, particularly in our blood vessels, such as the aorta.

According to Dr. Bjorksten, aluminum potentiates the formation of cross-linkages, causing blood vessels to become stiff and "hard," like old, dried-out garden hoses. Indeed, he has discovered a relationship between aluminum accumulation in tissues and death rates of the population at large. Aluminum levels are significantly lower in tissues of individuals who are active and aware in their 80s and 90s as compared with matched populations exhibiting the severe ravages of aging.

As previously noted, the original use of EDTA in the United States was for the treatment of heavy metal toxicity. It was applied to battery factory workers suffering from lead poisoning, a rare occurrence more than 30 years ago, but not so today.

Lead poisoning has become a major health threat. It has been established that we have 500 to 700 times more lead in our bones than our ancestors did. Those lead deposits, it appears, are released into our bloodstream under stress, following a severe trauma, or during a high fever from an infection, thus poisoning us most when our resistance is lowest.

No one is immune. The affluent person as well as the ghetto resident is at risk, as Dr. Vernon Houk, director of environmental health services at the Center for Disease Control in Atlanta pointed out. He said, "Lead toxicity is not, as once thought, confined to lower-income urban areas."

Lead is absorbed by eating, breathing, or through the skin. In previous years, concern primarily centered on lead ingestion via paint or industrial exposure. Today we have identified dozens of hazardous sources—atmospheric lead from smelters, coal, and leaded gasoline motor vehicle exhausts. The last accounts for half or more of the lead in our bodies.

If you eat vegetation grown by the roadside, drink milk, eat meat from animals grazing on our lead-contaminated pastures, or cook in improperly glazed pottery, you increase your exposure to lead. Moreover, there is absorbable lead in a bewildering variety of seemingly innocuous products: mascara, tobacco, curtain weights, newsprint, toothpaste, hair dyes, canned fruit and fruit juices, wine (with leaded caps), and some pesticides.

Subclinical exposure often results in subtle, yet significant, adverse health effects. In children, it manifests itself in behavioral problems, particularly hyperactivity and learning disabilities. In adults, relatively low levels may trigger headaches, digestive disorders, and general irritability.

Lead, like aluminum, is a potent catalyst of free radical reactions caused by peroxidation of unsaturated fatty acids. These metals, unlike the nutritional elements, have no "normal" site to bind them. They are always toxic, in more ways than one, since they greatly increase the rate of tissue degeneration from free radical damage.

If chelation did nothing more than eliminate lead from the body—and EDTA is in fact the recognized treatment of choice for this very problem—it would deserve the equivalent of a medical "Oscar."

Why? Because EDTA does much more than just get the lead out. It may be the answer to another of our most pressing health problems: reducing the incidence of cancer.

One piece of significant research, thus far ignored, was published in the scientific journal *Environment International* in 1980 by Swiss scientists from the Institute for Radiation Therapy and Nuclear Medicine at the University of Zurich.

In the course of earlier tests, Dr. W. Blumer and Dr. T. Reich found that the cancer mortality among 231 adult persons living adjacent to a heavily traveled highway was much higher than among persons living in a traffic-free section of the same town.

The authors postulated that the higher cancer mortality was due to automotive emissions as well as dust from "automobile roads," since they contain lead, cadmium, and other carcinogens. That speculation is supported by findings of a higher incidence of cancer deaths in cities than in the country, even among nonsmokers. Long-continued exposure to small amounts of lead can reduce resistance to the development of cancer.

Blumer and Reich are the only researchers to date to compare the subsequent death rates in a matched population of chelated and nonchelated persons. In the residential area in question, 59 of the adults living adjacent to the busy roadway received chelation therapy. One hundred seventy-two matched control subjects did not.

During the 18 years of follow-up, only one of the 59 chelated patients (1.7 percent) died of cancer; of the 172 persons not treated with EDTA, 30 (17 percent) died of cancer, or ten times more percentage wise. Try as they might, the investigators could find no factor other than chelation to explain the vast disparity in cancer mortality.

Their conclusion? Chelation was solely responsible for a 90 percent decrease in the incidence of cancer during the long-term follow-up. As for deaths from all other causes—cardiovascular disease included—overall mortality rates were significantly lower in the chelated group. A skeptical University of Zurich epidemiologist who examined the data confirmed the Blumer-Reich data.

Dr. Harry B. Demopoulos, associate professor of pathology at New York University Medical Center and an internationally known cancer researcher, has correlated heavy metal accumulation, free radical activity, and lipid peroxidation with the initiation and promotion of cancer.

New research from Japan introduces an entirely new anti-cancer aspect of EDTA. It was found that EDTA injected intravenously into mice increased the blood serum concentration of interferon four to twelvefold over the concentration induced by intravenous injections of lipopolysaccharides alone. This would explain why some patients feel so much better immediately upon being chelated. They could be suffering impaired immunity with symptoms relieved by the increased interferon production.

Chelating physicians cautiously avoid claims that chelation reverses the aging process, both because it is too difficult, complex, and expensive to prove, and because it might serve to further alienate our nonchelating colleagues.

One graphic example, however, of the relationship between uncontrolled free radical activity and accelerated aging is the genetic disease known as progeria, caused by the hereditary absence of free radical scavenging enzymes. Most TV viewers will remember having seen two victims of this heart-wrenching ailment when the cameras trailed them on a visit to Disneyland in 1983. Though neither had yet celebrated a tenth birthday, they resembled little old men. Typical progeria sufferers are wrinkled, have dried and sagging skin, are bald, bent, and have frail bodies crippled by arthritis and advanced cardiovascular disease before puberty. They usually die of "old age" while still in their teens. One form of progeria has been successfully treated by administering the free radical scavenging enzyme peroxidase.

Our biological time clock, which begins ticking at birth, seems to run at a speed determined by our body's efficiency in taking command of free radical chemical reactions. Reduced defenses against destructive free radical activity accelerate the aging process. Further evidence comes from the animal kingdom. Studies show that those mammals with the longest lifespans have the highest relative levels of SOD (superoxide dismutase), an anti-oxidant enzyme produced within the body.

As noted before, EDTA not only restricts free radical proliferation, but also allows the body's natural anti-oxidant defenses to regain control. Both are good reasons to accept EDTA chelation as a credible approach to healthful life extension.

And no discussion of all possible benefits of chelation therapy can be complete without mention of its potential for life extension. Research that has been going on for more than three decades has continually demonstrated that the lifespan of some very primitive organisms are dramatically extended when chelating agents are added to their culture medium. In some tests, increases of up to 50 percent the normal life span were recorded.

When distinguished gerontological researcher Dr. Johan Bjorksten reviewed and analyzed all the pertinent research and interpreted the data as it might apply to humans, he estimated the immediate widespread use of chelation therapy would result in mean lifespan increases of from 9 to 18 years for males and from 7 to 16 years for females.

To sum up the good news: We can *expect* chelation therapy to result in dramatic health improvements that go far beyond those linked directly to improved circulation. Bringing free radical reactions under control buys time—time for ailing cells to rebuild, time for rejuvenated cells to repair damaged tissue, time for diseased organs to heal.

Dr. Bjorksten considers it reasonable to hope for an ultimate 15 percent increase in lifespan when men and women are routinely chelated preventively early in life. Whether you are presently 15—or far older—being chelated offers you renewed hope for a substantially expanded high-quality lifespan.

8

Now, the Bad News: You'll Have to Foot the Bill

As of this writing, being chelated is much like having extraordinary beauty or great wealth—a rare and distinctive privilege to be enjoyed only by a relatively small, elite portion of the population.

If you are not related to a physician (many doctors are "closet chelators" who routinely chelate themselves and their loved ones but do not offer this treatment to patients), therapy is available only to those who can afford to pay for it—$3000 or thereabouts—out of their own pockets.

Even if you have the most comprehensive medical coverage, and thought yourself protected from every possible major or minor health problem, it is no go. Neither government nor private health insurance carriers will pay for the medical expenses of chelation therapy, except in rare instances.

When I say rare instances, I mean exactly that. Only a very few times in my many years of experience with hundreds of chelation patients have health insurers paid a claim. I remember them well, for in almost every instance, payment was some kind of fluke.

For example, the case of Mr. M., a patient who owned a business and paid large monthly medical insurance premiums for his more than 300 employees. When he developed atherosclerosis and opted for chelation therapy, his company's insurance carrier turned down his request for payment.

He didn't argue.

"No problem," he smiled, "I'll just cancel our policy and take the company business elsewhere."

His check arrived in the mail that week.

Then there was Mr. D, a man who held a senior position with a large, well-known health insurance firm, a company which, by the way, has routinely turned down chelation patients' claims. When this gentleman required chelating, having decided it was his best chance for recovery from a heart attack, he had no difficulty getting his claims paid. Easy for him. He authorized the signing of his own check!

And then there was the case of Mrs. K, a lovely lady, gentle and soft-spoken, but without such well-placed connections. Not knowing any better, she mailed her bills for chelation treatment off to Medicare and promptly received a check for $1600 by return mail. When she told me, I was dumbfounded.

"Oh, my," she enthused at her next visit, quite pleased. "You see, doctor, they do pay after all."

Two months later, she sent off an additional bill, for the next series of chelation treatments, with all the proper substantiating documents, and back came the more usual Medicare response: "We don't pay for that."

"But, you paid last time," she complained.

Obviously, some red-faced bureaucrat had goofed—and all she has received since have been demands to give the $1600 back.

On a few occasions, when their labor union leader had leverage with the insurance carrier and was willing to go to bat for them, coal miners have been reimbursed. And claims are sometimes paid by smaller, more obscure local-type insurance companies. It's my impression they are so far out of the mainstream, they don't know what chelation is.

That just about covers the exceptional circumstances under which you *might* have your chelation bills paid. You must be someone, know someone, or be gosh darn lucky. So be warned, the bad news about chelation is it is only going to hurt you in one place—the pocketbook.

You do have one more option. You can sue! And you'll probably win.

Litigious patients have on almost every occasion won judgments against insurance companies when they have been denied payment on frivolous grounds.

Courts have typically taken a dim view of attempts by insurance companies to deny a policyholder's payment for whatever medical treatment he prefers, as witness the judicial opinion written by Judge Francis N. Pecora of the City Court of New York City in the case of Brigitta Bruell against Associated Hospital Service of New York and United Medical Service, Inc.

Ruling against the health insurance companies that had refused payment to Mrs. Bruell because the treatment she selected was not FDA approved, the judge wrote: "Nowhere in the contract is the word 'necessary' treatment defined as a treatment which must be FDA approved. Moreover, implicit in contracts of this nature is the notion that a patient has a right to rely on his physician's decision as to what types of treatment are necessary for use against the patient's ill conditions.

"If the Defendant's (the insurance company's) position is upheld, which permits them to make value judgments as to correctness of judgment of duly licensed physicians, then the rights of the patients to such contracts will become highly subjective and will be determined at the whim and caprice of Defendants' medical advisory committee, whoever they may be.

"If medical coverage were to be denied each time an insurance company could provide a licensed physician to testify that, in his expert opinion, a treatment given by another licensed physician was not medically necessary or efficient, then no medical treatment could survive a denial of coverage."

In a similar case, Judge Paul Jones of Industrial Claims in Brevard County, Florida, ruled that the bills of Robert J. Rogers, M.D., be paid by the carrier, Continental National American Insurance, on behalf of the employee, Mr. Gerald Tillman.

Mr. Tillman, prior to consulting Dr. Rogers, had received extensive medical treatment, including several surgical procedures for reduction of back and leg pains, but continued to suffer. Only after receiving chelation therapy did he experience pain relief. Continental, however, denied payment. Judge Jones ruled for Mr. Tillman, stating Dr. Rogers's treatment of the patient with chelation therapy was "both reasonable and necessary and the employer/carrier should be responsible for the charges for treatment of the claimant in accordance with the standard medical fee schedule."

When the state of Florida, in a separate legal action, then attempted to restrict Dr. Rogers's chelation practice, the District Court of

Appeals ruled that the State Board of Medical Examiners was "without authority to deprive physicians' patients of their voluntary election to receive chelation therapy in treatment of arteriosclerosis simply because that mode of treatment had not received endorsement of the majority of the medical profession."

After lengthy hearings, Acting Chief Judge Boyer admonished those who had attempted to squash Dr. Rogers's practice of chelation, saying for the record: "History teaches us that virtually all progress in science and medicine has been accomplished as a result of the courageous efforts of those members of the profession willing to pursue their theories in the face of tremendous odds despite the criticism of fellow practitioners.

"Copernicus was thought to be a heretic when he theorized that the earth was not the center of the universe. Banishment and prison was the reward for discovering that the world was round. Pasteur was ridiculed for his theory that unseen organisms caused infection. Freud met only resistance and derision in pioneering the field of psychiatry.

"We can only wonder what would have been the condition of the world today and the field of medicine in particular had those in the midstream of their profession been permitted to prohibit continued treatment and thereby impede progress in those and other fields of science and the healing arts."

On August 27, 1982, the courts once again spoke out in defense of chelation. Medicare had refused to pay claims for *any* type of treatment for *any* patient who consulted Dr. Leo J. Bolles (a state of Washington medical doctor) for *any* reason, on the grounds that he offered services "not consistent with good medical practice." Dr. Bolles is a chelationist.

After two years of hearings, it was Judge Gordon McLean Callow's opinion that, "The record is replete with examples of dramatic improvement in some patients as a result of this unique strategy."

Commenting on the negative testimony about chelation that had been presented by the many anti-chelation physicians, the judge noted a "decided reluctance on the part of organized or established medicine to undertake further research on chelation therapy. In this writer's opinion, this reluctance borders, based on the evidence in this record, upon medical negligence."

Judge Callow classified the long and intensively fought court battle as, "another skirmish in the intense war between the medical 'establishment' and the medical 'mavericks,' for want of more polite descriptions." And expressing admiration for the "maverick" physicians who had testified in favor of chelation therapy, he offered this opinion:

"While I do not believe the undercurrent allegation that the medical establishment is against chelation therapy because of its possible impact on the current $20,000 bill attached to each heart bypass surgery, the sometimes overtly arrogant approach taken by certain of the government's witnesses in this case toward any possibility that the 'chelationists' might be on to something is only otherwise explicable on the supposition that the medical 'establishment,' including the pharmaceutical houses, are unwilling to experiment with EDTA unless huge monetary rewards await."

The judge concluded, "If these men are right in their obviously honest convictions (and they may be), the medical profession owes at least a portion of its enormous research resources to a fair and objective trial of chelation therapy in the treatment of vascular disease, obviously a major physical problem in American society."

Hopeful as these victories are for those patients who turn to the courts, there is a "Catch 22" aspect to seeking judicial relief via a breach of contract suit against your health insurer. Even if you win, you lose, inasmuch as you will most likely incur $10,000 or more in court and legal costs to secure a $2000 to $3000 reimbursement.

In one spectacular example, a wealthy patient, able to pursue the issue on principle, fought in the courts for almost five years, at an out-of-pocket cost of more than $15,000, before he 'won' a $2750 judgment.

The way things now stand, I advise chelation patients that they can come out ahead by *not* submitting their bills for chelation treatments to their insurance carriers. Once insurers get wind that bills are in any way associated with chelation, they will refuse to pay for the initial physical exam and all other tests that make up the prechelation protocol. When tied to chelation, more often than not, claims for reimbursement of those bills are also turned down, and the patient loses the $400 to $500 he would otherwise have collected.

Hard to believe? Perhaps. But fact all the same. When people learn that their health insurance will not cover chelation treatments, they are initially stunned. Then come the questions.

"Is chelation legal?"

"Why won't they pay?"

"What's going on?"

First things first. Chelation therapy is completely legal. Doctors who provide this treatment as warranted are not operating on the fringe. Nor are they violating any state, Federal, or local statutes, or acting contrary to the highest medical ethics. State and Federal courts have repeatedly reaffirmed a licensed physician's freedom to use any procedure or drug which, in his considered judgment, is to the best interest of his patient.

The American Medical Association's position on this issue is equally clear. In response to a query on the question of the legality of chelation therapy, Dr. Asher J. Finkel (Scientific Activities Division, AMA, Chicago) wrote, "We (the AMA) have always maintained that any licensed physician is free to use any drug approved by the FDA for marketing, in any way the physician deems appropriate in his best clinical judgment. If your physician believes in the usefulness of chelation therapy, for whatever purpose in his clinical judgment, he is perfectly free to use it."

If legality is not at issue, what is?

At a time when 71 percent of medical expenses in this country are paid by third-party insurers, how are Medicare, Blue Cross, and other insurance companies able to refuse payment for chelation?

As in many other situations where ordinary citizens are forced into "go fight City hall" wrangles with huge, impersonal organizations, when you trace the problem to the source, you usually find bungled legislation or bureaucratic distortion of legislated guidelines. So it is here.

To understand what has been happening, a brief explanation of Medicare is necessary. The Federal medical insurance program for people 65 and older was passed into law in 1965 under the Social Security Act. It consists of two parts:

Part A: Hospital insurance—covers all eligible persons and is funded by compulsory contributions out of workers' wages and payments by their employers.

Part B: Medical insurance—supplementary and optional, for persons 65 and older who pay a modest monthly premium for approximately 80 percent (or less, in most cases) reimbursement based on "allowable charges" for doctors' and surgeons' fees and other medical services not included under Part A. Part B Medicare reimbursement is administered by private health insurance companies that are paid with taxpayer dollars to scrutinize payment requests and weed out the fraudulent or excessive.

When Medicare contractors refuse payment for chelation, they are following official guidelines from Washington that state that "EDTA chelation therapy is a covered service only if administered for: emergency treatment of hypercalcemia, control of ventricular arrhythmias and heart block secondary to digitalis toxicity, or (with another form of EDTA) for lead poisoning."

The guidelines were prepared with the help of government scientists and physicians who have little or no experience with chelation, or have come to an adverse judgment without a careful study of the actual hard scientific data, or are representatives of a competing specialty such as cardiovascular surgery.

According to Medicare protocol, chelation therapy is not "medically indicated and necessary" for the treatment of atherosclerosis, and therefore does not meet "accepted standards of medical practice." They have labeled chelation "experimental" because "there is a lack of well-designed, controlled clinical trials of its effectiveness, and that the risks to health and safety are a cause for concern."

Do these instructions to Medicare contractors to deny coverage for chelation therapy for atherosclerosis represent a sincere and honest attempt to protect the gullible from the danger of an unproven treatment? You be the judge.

While we shall cover the issue of EDTA's safety more thoroughly in another chapter, keep in mind that multiple studies, as well as three decades of clinical experience with hundreds of thousands of patients, have demonstrated the treatment to be safe when properly administered.

Experimental? With more than 400,000 people having taken more than 6 million chelation treatments to date?

Let's consider "medically indicated and necessary." Imagine the response to that one from men and women, now recovered, who turned to chelation as a last resort.

It is all too clear that the difficulties lie not with chelation, but with the way the Medicare statutes were written, and are being interpreted. There can be no doubt that congressional intent, under the general provisions of the Medicare statute, was for the treating physician, together with his or her patient, to be the primary determinant of what is "medically indicated and necessary" treatment and care.

Congress also included in the Medicare statute a provision *guaranteeing* patients free choice among health service providers, indicating their steadfast resolve not to interfere with the normal patient/physician relationship, nor to allow a Medicare carrier to override that professional medical judgment made by a competent physician in good faith.

It is when you examine the "proven effectiveness" challenge that it becomes obvious that patients' health insurance rights are being violated, for Medicare and its contract administrators are demanding a higher order of proof of both safety and efficacy for chelation therapy than for just about every other accepted-for-payment treatment, such as coronary bypass and vascular surgery.

In 1972, the United States Congress passed legislation establishing the Office of Technological Assessment (OTA) to help the government study and assess emerging technologies. In 1978, in response to a congressional request for an evaluation of the usual and customary medical practices in this country, OTA submitted a report entitled, "Efficacy and Safety of Medical Technologies," with this startling conclusion: "ONLY TEN TO TWENTY PERCENT OF ALL PROCEDURES CURRENTLY USED IN MEDICAL PRACTICE HAVE BEEN SHOWN TO BE EFFICACIOUS BY CONTROLLED TRIAL."

Close scrutiny of the 133-page document reveals a decided antichelation therapy bias involved in the way payment guidelines are applied. Health insurance carriers have routinely, without question, shelled out billions for treatments never subjected to controlled clinical trials, and never proven beneficial.

The OTA was highly critical of (among other procedures) coronary bypass surgery, pointing out this procedure had become the primary approach to treatment of coronary artery disease, with as many as 70,000 such surgeries performed each year, at an annual costs of more than $1 billion (that figure rose to $2 billion in 1982), despite there having never been clearly demonstrated benefits over nonsurgical treatments. The report singled out coronary bypass surgery as an example of widely used technologies that "have been diffused rapidly before careful evaluation," adding, "Claims that the operation prevents death remain largely unproven."

As for the procedures that have been tested by controlled trial, it was the conclusion of the OTA study that even those formal studies which had been completed and published are of questionable value, inasmuch as careful review of research reports in leading publications revealed that more than 75 percent had invalid or insupportable conclusions as a result of statistical problems alone. The fact is that few clinical trials are well-enough designed to yield valuable results.

"Personal experience," the report suggests, "is perhaps the oldest and most common informal method of judging the efficacy and safety of a medical technology."

Precisely. Witness the personal experience of the hundreds of chelating physicians who each and every day see the best evidence of all that they are using an effective treatment—recovered patients.

Following the government's lead, private health insurance companies have taken the stance, "What Medicare won't pay for, we won't either." Blue Cross/Blue Shield, as a matter of fact, has a published "hit list" of nonreimbursable procedures (hyperbaric oxygen for stroke, hair analysis for toxic metal poisoning, and chelation therapy for atherosclerosis are among them). And these decisions are heartily endorsed by professional associations biased against competing procedures.

"Surely," patients say, "things will eventually change. The government (and the insurance industry) can't hold out forever."

I wouldn't bet on it because it's a matter of bucks.

If the truth be known, the government can't afford the payments it's already committed to, much less take on new obligations. The looming Medicare crisis has Congress hard-pressed to find ways to cut services, not add new ones.

Let's assume for a moment that the government has a change of heart. Medicare and the health insurance industry agree to pick up the tab for chelation therapy.

The first year or so, the savings would be substantial. If only one-fourth of the 110,000 persons annually undergoing vascular surgery (a $30,000+ procedure) chose chelation instead (at a cost of roughly $3000), health insurers would save a minimum of $750 million.

Why then so much resistance? Perhaps they have looked further down the line. Perhaps they are not as oblivious to chelation therapy's benefits and potential as they pretend to be. As chelation experts are all too well aware, the therapy is needed by far more people than those already in so sorry a condition that they are candidates for surgery. How many more? That is the trillion dollar question.

No one knows for sure how many potential chelation patients are out there, but we do have figures upon which we can make an educated estimate.

What percentage of our entire population has serious atherosclerosis? Over 50 percent of the deaths in this country are caused by circulatory ailments related to arterial disease. If paid-for chelation were available to just those already exhibiting symptoms (this usually happens five to ten years prior to death), we are talking about chelating about 30 million people for a total cost of $90 billion. A mind-boggling figure.

But what about all those men and women without symptoms? A study conducted during the Korean and Vietnam wars on autopsies of American soldiers revealed arterial plaque formation in the majority of these seemingly healthy young men. Improved diagnostic techniques, such as nuclear magnetic resonance, total body CAT scans, digital subtraction angiography, and gray zone ultrasound imaging, will soon be detecting developing atherosclerotic disease in almost every adult man and woman (and many boys and girls over the age of puberty). Now we are talking about 100 million chelation candidates, and the cost would be equivalent to a third of the Federal budget in 1984.

Is Medicare (and the health insurance industry) determined to save you or themselves? The health insurance industry is in trouble. They are in business to make money, to pay dividends to stockholders. That is tough to do at a time when health care costs are skyrocketing faster than higher premiums can be charged. Give them any excuse to duck payments, and they will do it.

As U.S. Senator Edward Kennedy said, "To the (health) insurance companies, people are the enemy, because every private claim is a threat to corporate profit."

It is no secret that the government is already struggling with the biggest budget deficits in its history, that Social Security is in deep trouble (mainly because more people are living longer than originally anticipated), and that Medicare is an almost bankrupt system.

Government economists estimate the Medicare fund will be more than $1 trillion in the red by the year 2005. Medicare payments are rising faster than revenues in the system's Hospital Insurance Trust Fund, not only because of rising health care costs and the proliferation of medical services, but because there are growing numbers of elderly citizens enjoying longer lifespans.

Unpleasant as it is to think of our government as making decisions that favor economics over lives, such may actually be the case.

In 1973, Alexander Leaf, then head of the President's Scientific Commission on Aging, publicly stated, "To consider any extension of the human lifespan without a serious effort to anticipate and plan for the impact of increased longevity on society would be entirely irresponsible."

To sum up, the good news about chelation is that it probably will help you live longer. The bad news is that health insurers, the Social Security Administration, and Medicare probably can't afford to have that happen.

9

Harvard Snubs Chelation

Mr. K., a married 58-year-old fabrication plant manager, first discovered he was a candidate for vascular surgery when he checked in for a series of tests after having suffered leg and chest pains.

Since the K.'s are New York City residents, with easy access to the finest medical care and the most highly trained specialists, they were determined not to accept a first opinion, even coming from an impressive cardiologist associated with one of New York's leading university-affiliated hospitals.

Mrs. K., well read and inquisitive, embarked on an intensive, month-long search of the medical and popular literature relevant to Mr. K.'s disease, and discovered chelation.

"Let's ask the doctor," Mr. K. said, never too quick to share his wife's enthusiasms. They did.

His response: "I don't know anything about it, except that it's no good and dangerous."

A scientific evaluation? Hardly.

An extraordinary response? All too common.

Although few well-trained professionals would be so brazen as to admit in the same breath that they are commenting on something about which they have little or no knowledge, the average physician who objects to chelation is equally ill-informed, but just hides it better. Establishment medicine has long broadcast unfounded objections to chelation therapy, warning of documented dangers, for which there is little basis in fact.

To anyone contemplating chelation, such warnings arouse much distress. As a matter of fact, they caused my publisher understandable concern. Just prior to contracting for this book, Mr. Sol Stein, president of Stein and Day Publishers, received the January 1983 issue of *The Harvard Medical School Health Letter*, denouncing chelation therapy for heart disease as an unproven medical treatment with clear evidence that it may be harmful.

With his permission, I will make you privy to our correspondence.

First, the communication the publisher received from my alma mater:

> Chelation therapy for heart disease: Hundreds of physicians or clinics in the United States provide so-called chelation therapy in an attempt to open narrowed blood vessels in the heart. In the usual treatment program, a chemical known as EDTA is injected intravenously for one to two hours. The patient then rests for a few days, and the treatment is repeated from 5 to as many as 50 times. After weeks to months, at a cost of about $3,000, the patient is supposed to have better circulation to the heart, with a lowered risk of heart attack and fewer symptoms (such as pain or breathlessness).
>
> The rationale for this treatment is that EDTA binds calcium and removes it from the bloodstream. Because calcium is found in the plaques that obstruct diseased arteries, proponents of chelation hope that lowering blood levels of calcium will allow calcium to dissolve out of the plaques, causing them to grow smaller. But, in fact, (1) the bulk of the material in a plaque is fiber, not calcium; (2) EDTA has not been proven to remove the calcium from plaques; (3) and, to date, no persuasive evidence from properly controlled studies has established that chelation therapy relieves symptoms.
>
> An overdose of EDTA, rapidly administered, is potentially lethal. If given slowly, the drug is relatively harmless, although it can produce kidney damage. Temporary discomfort of one sort or another can also occur.
>
> Chelation therapy does have established value as a treatment for heavy-metal poisoning, but it has not proven itself in heart disease. Anyone who accepts chelation therapy is automatically a "guinea pig," and unless the treatment is given as part of a carefully controlled trial, he or she is a guinea pig without purpose, as no useful information is going to be obtained.*

---

*Excerpted from the January 1983 issue of *The Harvard Medical School Health Letter* © 1983 President and Fellows of Harvard College.

On January 6, 1983, the publisher wrote me the following letter:

> I was concerned to see the January 1983 *Harvard Medical School Health Letter* refer to chelation therapy on its front page as an "unproven medical treatment." I am much less concerned with their comments about an overdose being potentially lethal because an overdose of aspirin and a hell of a lot of other things are potentially lethal. I have some concern about the possibility of kidney damage but the major concern is with the fact that they say in the second paragraph that "to date, no persuasive evidence from properly controlled studies has established that chelation therapy relieves symptoms."
>
> I'd welcome hearing your reaction at the earliest.

The following morning, I spoke with Mr. Stein by phone. Our conversation was cordial, but to the point. He wanted to make certain that he would not be irresponsibly publishing material that might cause public harm. He made it clear that publication of this book hinged on my drafting a letter with supporting documentation to answer the questions raised in the *Harvard Medical School Health Letter*. He also informed me he intended to correspond with the editors of the *Health Letter*, and was going to use my letter and my supporting documents to challenge their statements.

Fair enough. I had met a tough, but open-minded judge. It took me more than two weeks to draft my reply. On January 26th I wrote:

> Dear Mr. Stein:
>
> I am writing in answer to your questions concerning EDTA chelation therapy in the treatment of occlusive arterial disease. More specifically, I will point out what I consider to be errors in the January 1983 *Harvard Medical School Health Letter* (HMSHL). I am dismayed but not surprised that such a prestigious health letter, carrying an implied endorsement of the medical school from which I graduated, could be so misinformed about this safe and effective alternative to bypass surgery and to other treatments.
>
> With the exception of occasional use in life-threatening cardiac irregularities caused by digitalis toxicity, or in the rare treatment of dangerously high blood calcium, I doubt whether contributors to the HMSHL have had sufficient personal experience to criticize

EDTA chelation therapy. They seem unaware that it is the "disodium" form of EDTA which is used in the treatment of atherosclerosis, as distinguished form the "calcium-disodium" form used in the treatment of heavy metal poisoning.

There exists a difference of opinion between experts and, in this instance, I believe that I am far more expert in the use of EDTA chelation therapy than are contributors to the HMSHL. In addition to having been awarded my M.D. degree from Harvard Medical School, I am board certified as a specialist by both the American Board of Family Practice and the American Board of Chelation Therapy. I am presently Vice President of the American Academy of Medical Preventics, a professional association of physicians who endorse chelation therapy. I have been using EDTA in the treatment of occlusive arterial disease for approximately ten years, with marked and lasting benefit in 75 to 95 percent of hundreds of patients treated. Observed benefits have correlated with the total number of treatments. No harm has come to any of those patients as a result of EDTA therapy.

The HMSHL states, ". . . proponents of chelation hope that lowering blood levels of calcium will allow calcium to dissolve out of the plaques, causing them to grow smaller." Any such assertion is oversimplified and misrepresents the position of well-trained, chelating physicians. There is no evidence that chelation cherapy reduces plaque size in humans. On the other hand, there is a wealth of evidence that the symptoms of reduced blood flow improve in more than 75 percent of patients treated.

Published research also indicates that treatment with EDTA improves the efficiency of energy metabolism independently of any effects on blood flow.

The HMSHL further states that EDTA is injected intravenously for "one or two hours." No physician qualified in the proper use of EDTA would infuse a therapeutic dose at such a rapid rate. Three hours is considered the minimum safe duration for an infusion. More rapid infusions have been responsible for kidney changes. Any medicine given in too high a dose over too short a time can cause harm.

The HMSHL correctly states that the therapy may last from weeks to months at a cost of about $3000. They neglect, however, to point out that bypass surgery usually costs from seven to ten times that amount with a significant incidence of death, pain, suffering, and other serious complications, including long-term disability. Chelation therapy, properly administered, incurs no such risks. The cost of other nonsurgical treatments can also equal or exceed the cost of chelation therapy over the same period of time. Cost figures must be considered in that perspective.

The HMSHL states that "... no persuasive evidence from properly controlled studies has established that chelation therapy relieves symptoms." Physicians advocating chelation therapy are faced with a double standard. Bypass surgery was enthusiastically accepted without any such controlled studies. Coronary artery bypass has never been proven by "properly controlled studies" to be other than placebo effect. In fact, there is another operation called cardiac sympathectomy which interrupts nerves that stimulate the heart with adrenalinlike substances. Cardiac sympathectomy also improves symptoms. It is impossible to perform bypass surgery without also interrupting sympathetic nerves, reducing spasm of coronary arteries and reducing workload of the heart. It has never been proven in "properly controlled studies" which effect is most important, bypass or sympathectomy.

Enclosed are nine recently published scientific papers concerning chelation therapy [readers will find these referenced and described in greater detail at the end of chapter 16, Take This to Your Doctor], three of which show statistically significant, objective measurements of improved blood flow following EDTA chelation. The study by Dr. Casdorph on heart disease might be criticized because changes in cardiac ejection fraction were relatively small. Statistical analysis in that paper was based solely on the probability of measuring 17 improvements in 18 patients, irrespective of the degree of improvement. This is analogous to calculating the probability of flipping a coin 18 consecutive times and getting 17 heads. It is not necessary to consider the degree of change of cardiac ejection fraction to prove a high degree of statistical significance. Observed clinical improvement was also dramatic. Dr. Casdorph's second study, which measures brain blood flow, contains even more convincing data to prove that EDTA chelation therapy results in a very significant improvement in circulation to the brain. The probability that these results could have been due to random chance are less than five in ten thousand. That study was duplicated and confirmed independently by other researchers using a different technology.

A manuscript in press by Drs. Casdorph and Farr does not offer statistical proof of effectiveness, but that paper does describe four patients who had each been told to have a leg amputated. They sought out chelation instead and all four are now enjoying a good quality of life, able to walk on both legs without the recommended amputations.

Another study reports the results of kidney function tests done on 383 consecutive patients, before and after treatment with EDTA for chronic degenerative disease. That study showed no adverse effects from EDTA, and it did show a statistically significant improvement in kidney function following chelation. One patient, of the 383 studied, was at first an exception. She was an 86-year-old woman who began the treatments with preexisting abnormal kidney function and experienced further deterioration following EDTA. Three months following treatment her kidney function was closer to normal than when she began. Physicians qualified to administer intravenous EDTA give reduced dosages at less frequent intervals to patients with diminished kidney function.

One enclosure is a review of the scientific literature concerning kidney effects of EDTA. That review indicates that reports of kidney damage stem from patients with preexisting kidney disease prior to EDTA or who suffered with diseases frequently associated with primary kidney disorders. Also, during the early use of EDTA the dose-rate of administration was often six or more times higher than is now considered safe.

Temporary discomfort from EDTA mentioned in the HMSHL is quite minimal when compared with the discomfort of bypass surgery or even coronary artery angiograms.

The HMSHL reference to "guinea pigs" prompts a similar observation that anyone who accepts bypass surgery is also "automatically a guinea pig." Why is it that the critics of chelation should demand that millions of dollars be spent in large-scale, double-blind, controlled studies of chelation to prove that the benefits are not due to placebo effect, while at the same time they enthusiastically refer patients for bypass surgery for which no similar studies exist? The proponents of bypass surgery say that they do not need controlled studies to prove effectiveness because the benefits are so obvious. It is equally obvious to practitioners of chelation therapy that their patients also improve, for far less cost and at very little risk.

Critics of chelation therapy say that it is "unproven," but they ignore the fact that no funds have been made available for research with chelation. Committees that control government research funds seem to share a common bias with the critics. These same committees have allocated tens of millions of dollars toward research of bypass surgery while experts are still arguing about whether medical therapy might not be equally effective in many or most patients subjected to surgery.

The three statistically significant studies that I have described might still be criticized because they are not double-blind. These studies were performed at the personal expense of physicians in practice, using patients as their own controls. That is, objective measurements were made on patients prior to therapy and follow-up measurements were made after therapy. Critics of chelation therapy may say that since both the patient and the treating physician knew that every patient was receiving EDTA, the observed benefits would be in the range of what one might expect from the placebo effect. With 75 to 90 percent of patients improving and with symptoms which had often not responded to all other available therapies, it is not likely that the placebo effect could be responsible for such universal benefit.

I consider the enclosed reports to be good science. All scientific observations begin with anecdotal reports and then with a small series of patients, prior to undertaking the very expensive, large-scale, double-blind studies in which half of the patients truly are "guinea pigs," and unknowingly do not receive the active ingredient under study.

Contributors to the HMSHL seem to be relying on outdated reports published ten to fifteen years ago for their opinions. I doubt that they are aware of the recently published data which I have cited. Human Sciences Press, publisher of the *Journal of Holistic Medicine,* in which six of the nine enclosures have appeared, informs me that the Francis A. Countway Library of Medicine at Harvard Medical School does receive the *Journal of Holistic Medicine* and that it should have been available to the HMSHL staff. In defense of the HMSHL, I might add that these recent papers would be somewhat difficult to find since the *Journal of Holistic Medicine* is not yet listed in the *Index Medicus,* nor are papers published in that journal available for a computer search on the topic of chelation therapy. The *Journal of Holistic Medicine* applied to the National Library of Medicine two years ago for listing in the *Index Medicus* and for availability to the MEDLINE computer search program. A committee which selects journals for such listings can approve only ten or fifteen percent of all publications received by the National Library of Medicine. Monetary and personnel limitations do not allow for a more comprehensive service. Many foreign language publications are not received by the National Library of Medicine and are therefore not even considered. A number of foreign research papers quite favorable to chelation therapy are in that category, and are listed as references in the enclosures. Most health care professionals are quite unaware that when they request a computer search on a specific topic they receive a representation of less than ten percent of what has been published in the world's scientific literature.

Experts with extensive experience in the use of chelation therapy routinely observe dramatic improvement in the vast majority of their patients and they do not feel justified in withholding this treatment if symptoms are present. The economics and medical politics of the situation are such that proponents of other therapies, especially bypass surgery and expensive prescription drugs, find themselves in a much more powerful position than that of chelating physicians. Big money and huge industries are involved. As chelation therapy is increasingly brought to public awareness, criticism from these more politically powerful sectors becomes stronger. The recent HMSHL is just one such example.

Approximately the same number of patients have undergone chelation therapy as have undergone bypass surgery. Most such patients have accepted chelation therapy on the recommendation of friends or family members who have previously been helped by chelation, despite the absence of insurance reimbursement and without benefit of the widespread media publicity and "status" associated with bypass surgery. They often chose chelation against the advice of their personal physicians and cardiologists. Chelation therapy is made available by physicians courageous enough to resist peer pressure and to provide a nontraditional treatment that they feel is safer and more effective.

To be completely fair, all forms of therapy should eventually be researched on equal terms. There is an urgent need for grant funding from the National Institutes of Health to allow proper studies to further prove or disprove safety and effectiveness of all therapies. EDTA is not patentable and a pharmaceutical company could not recover the research costs of such a study. Practicing physicians cannot afford to do more than limited studies. That leaves only NIH as a source of funding for an "orphan" type drug; that is, a drug which has been around for so long that the patent has expired and for which an important new use is discovered.

I sincerely doubt whether the best interests of the American public are being served by existing health care procedures and policies.

Sincerely,
Elmer M. Cranton, M.D.

The most immediate result of this interchange of letters was the contract for this book. But, on June 5, 1983, came a different, rather unexpected response from another quarter.

I received a letter from an influential Harvard alumnus who works closely with a Harvard Medical School dean. He wrote to tell me of his particular personal interest in chelation and in my rebuttal of the negative report in the HMSHL. He mentioned he had a quadruple arterial bypass three and one half years ago, and is good friends with a Texas physician and former classmate who happens to be one of the pioneers of chelation therapy in the United States.

Thinking he might one day benefit from chelation, he had communicated with the dean at Harvard to request they send him all the scientific material—research and test results—which had served as a source for the HMSHL chelation report.

"Only very recently," he wrote, "did I get the material requested. It was a copy of an article that had appeared in the *Internal Medicine News* of September 14th, written by a staff writer, Mr. W. R. Kubetin. The article quotes the opinions of doctors Harrison and Frommer and others. It is not a scientific paper of course but a popular rendition of opinions of others who may or may not have been involved with the chelation procedure. I was somewhat disappointed that the *Harvard Letter* would not investigate primary medical and scientific sources before printing its report."

One thing he might have mentioned, but did not, was the biased way in which the HMSHL staff chose to quote sources from the news tabloid. They carefully included all the anti-chelation comments, and just as carefully refrained from including any of the pro-chelation opinions.

This will not, of course, put an end to groundless anti-chelation charges, but it should serve notice to biased critics that they had better start doing their homework.

10

The Real Dangers You Haven't Been Warned About

Heard from your doctor lately? Has he called to check up on how you and your family are doing, or let you in on the latest news from his medical society? Does he keep tabs on you to make sure you don't inadvertently stumble into medical trouble? No?

If you live in Lincolnton, North Carolina, you get a very special type of personal medical service. You don't need to subscribe to the *Harvard Medical School Health Letter* to be misinformed about the dangers of chelation therapy. All you need do is make an appointment to visit a chelating physician.

At least that was Bobby Campbell's experience. Two days after he called my office and scheduled a visit, he received the following *unsolicited* communication (a Xeroxed document from the Council of Scientific Affairs of the American Medical Association) postmarked July 12, 1983, from John R. Gamble, Jr., M.D., a Lincolnton physician. It read:

> SUBJECT: Chelation Therapy
>
> QUESTION: How safe and effective is chelation therapy with ethylenediamine tetraacetic acid or its sodium salt for the treatment of atherosclerotic vascular disease?
>
> ANSWER: There was a consensus among all respondents that chelation therapy with ethylenediamine tetraacetic acid or its sodium salt was not an established treatment for atherosclerotic vascular disease.
>
> The original thesis that repeated intravenous infusions of the chelating agent, EDTA disodium, was of benefit to patients with

> coronary artery disease, as manifested by the anginal syndrome, has not been established in any well-designed, controlled trial. Although some uncontrolled studies claim positive benefits, others have shown no significant effects from such therapy. There is no supporting evidence that it has any significant effect upon the atherosclerotic plaque.
>
> Furthermore, the safety of using EDTA, especially in patients with coronary artery disease, is questionable. Chelation of plasma calcium will decrease the levels of ionized calcium and result in tetany, cardiac arrhythmias, convulsions, and respiratory arrest. It can cause renal tubular necrosis and renal failure, permanent renal damage, bone marrow depression, and prolongation of the prothrombin time.
>
> The majority of the respondents felt that this treatment was unacceptable or indeterminate therapy for atherosclerotic vascular disease. About half as many felt that it could still be considered investigational, i.e. worthy of a controlled trial under protocol.

At the bottom of the page: "The above response is provided as a service of the American Medical Association. It is based on current scientific and clinical information and does not represent endorsement by the AMA of particular diagnostic and therapeutic procedures or treatment."

And what did this prestigious organization cite as its reference? You guessed it. Outdated and incomplete reviews, composed primarily of editorial opinion by physicians with little or no chelation experience.

In Corpus Christi, Texas, a group of physicians, equally eager to warn the public of potential danger, banded together in a mass media approach. On July 29, 1983, the following advertisement, without mention of a sponsoring organization, but with an alphabetical listing of 247 doctors, appeared in the local daily, the *Corpus Caller*:

> MEDICAL NOTICE—The undersigned doctors agree that there is no good scientific evidence for any benefit from Chelation Therapy for heart disease or hardening of the arteries. Furthermore, it is probably of no value in that type of illness. It is worthy for the public to note that this method of treatment has not been approved by the FDA.

What was going on in Corpus Christi?

Curious, we began calling physicians listed, in alphabetical order. Of the first 11 contacted, only two were available to discuss their anti-chelation position.

Both referred us to Jean Oliver, at the Nueces County Medical Society, explaining they knew very little about it (the ad or chelation), but stated that "it" (chelation) was of "no value" and "dangerous."

Although each of these physicians was noticeably reluctant to speak to the issue, the first said he felt the "danger would be to make the patient believe that he is getting cured of something that has not been proved." The second doctor explained that EDTA takes calcium "out of the bones and everywhere else," but "probably does not take it out of arteries. . . . You could get osteoporosis, weakness in the bones, lose most of your strength out of your skeleton, and suffer bone pains."

When we called the offices of the Nueces County Medical Society, Mrs. Oliver denied the society had placed the ad and suggested we call Dr. Mario Eugenio, president of the group. Finally we reached Dr. Eugenio.

What was happening in Corpus Christi relative to chelation therapy?

"There have been a few problems."

"What kind of problems?"

"I am not in a position to tell you."

At the last, Dr. Eugenio offered the following: "There are some doctors using it, and charging $3000, and even wives are complaining their husbands are spending the money that they should be giving in the house for a treatment that would not be acceptable. That's what started us looking around."

But, if we really wanted to understand the "best positions" on the dangers involved with chelation, he suggested we go "right to the source" and contact the American Medical Association.

Although there is little doubt it is more dangerous to drive to the doctor's office than to be chelated once you get there, there are risks, and everyone considering chelation should be aware of them.

With more than 30 years of documented clinical experience with EDTA to guide them, chelating physicians today have access to valuable information unavailable to their predecessors when it comes to taking every possible precaution to safeguard patients against the possibility of injury.

Even so, it is quite possible that chelation therapy has resulted in unpredictable harm in some isolated instances because of the unusual idiosyncracies of individual patients. Without being facetious, there are citings in the medical literature of individuals so superallergic that they have died eating a peanut butter sandwich. The odds of such an occurrence are probably one in 50 million, but there are people who have had unfavorable reactions to almost any substance you can think of, peanuts included.

To the best of my knowledge and experience, it is extremely rare that a person is so allergic that he cannot be safely chelated, provided proper precautions are taken. When a patient does have an allergic reaction, it is rarely serious, and can be immediately counteracted or neutralized by a physician who is trained and knows what he is doing. In my experience, in just about every such instance, the sensitivity has not been to EDTA, but to one or more of the ingredients we add to the intravenous solution (vitamins and minerals, for example), which are manufactured with preservatives. When we detect a patient with allergies, we prepare a modified EDTA solution, custom-tailoring the ingredients to the individual sensitivity.

The EDTA solution includes some sodium, and there may be a potential hazard for patients whose cardiac status is precarious (borderline heart failure or heart failure controlled by medication). In those cases, where there is the danger that the infusion of fluid and salt can temporarily worsen a patient's condition, we carefully regulate diuretics, run the infusion much more slowly, space the treatments further apart, and monitor all aspects extremely carefully. With those precautions, most of the patients can still be chelated.

For many years it was thought that people with arrested tuberculosis should not be chelated because calcification of the tuberculoma is one factor believed to keep the disease in remission and from spreading. Now we know that EDTA's effect on that type of calcium is so minimal that there is only the remotest possibility of dissolving the calcium out of the calcium-coated granuloma in the lung wall. There have been no documented cases of this ever happening. But, just to be certain, we do serial chest x-rays on patients with a history of arrested tuberculosis.

Another worry that has proved unjustified over time is that patients with calcium kidney stones might be adversely effected if the EDTA partially dissolved the stones, which might then be dislodged and get trapped in the lower urinary passages leading to the bladder. This is only a potential risk in someone who has a large stone upstream, where the base of the kidney has a big open cavity. In such cases, of course, the kidney stone could be dislodged and cause a blockage to kidney drainage at any time, with or without chelation. Surgery may then be needed.

Kidney stones of some specific types may be dissolved by EDTA. There have been cases reported where, after long, long courses of repeated chelation therapy, they were not only partially dissolved, but then passed safely. In most instances, whether one has kidney stones or not has little bearing on the safety of being chelated.

One more bugaboo that deserves burying is the worry that EDTA impacting on calcified arteries might unseat plaque and unloose chunks that would eventually block smaller downstream blood vessels. Plaque dislodgement is always a danger in patients with such atherosclerosis. But the fact is, it has never been a documented complication of chelation therapy when administered in currently accepted doses and rates—a remarkable history in light of the enormous number of patients treated over the years.

There is some small possibility of EDTA chelation resulting in temporarily diminished kidney function, but only under very specific circumstances. If EDTA is administered too rapidly or in too large a dose for the patient's tolerance, the excreted toxic wastes can overload the kidneys, leading to impaired function. This is reversible if detected early and further chelation treatments delayed. If undetected and repeated chelations are administered, it could cause permanent kidney failure. The individual could spend the rest of his life on renal dialysis. It has happened. Your best protection is to be absolutely certain the doctor you choose knows what he is doing. (More on this later.)

To put this in proper perspective, be reminded that there is no medicine known to man that cannot cause harm if too much is given too fast. Every physician knows that.

Digitalis, for instance, used routinely for heart conditions, has a long half-life, meaning it stays in a patient's system so long, it is easy to overdose. The difference between a therapeutic and toxic dose is so small, a borderline dose can turn out to be lethal. One of the most unforgettable things I was told at medical school was that there is hardly a doctor alive who uses digitalis-type medicines to any extent who hasn't killed a patient with an inadvertent overdose.

What is true of every other medicinal substance is also true of EDTA, except that it has very low toxicity when compared with most other medicines. It has a half-life of less than one hour and is rapidly excreted unmetabolized. It has a remarkable safety record. After three decades of use in the United States, involving in excess of 400,000 patients and more than 6 million treatments, it has triggered fewer untoward effects than aspirin.

What better evidence than the notable absence of malpractice claims against chelating physicians? A thorough search of available case law data conducted both by students at the Georgetown University Law School and the National Association of Insurance Commissioners failed to turn up *any* reported legal actions involving the use of chelation for atherosclerosis.

Considering the controversial nature of chelation and the large number of treatments that have been given, it is indeed noteworthy that chelating physicians have not been subjected to the medical malpractice suits that have plagued their more traditional colleagues.

There have probably been some kidney failures—even kidney deaths—with chelation therapy, but to the best of my knowledge this always happened when the doctors gave too much, too fast, to patients already at peril because of compromised kidney function. To condemn chelation therapy because there have been careless applications by underqualified physicians is tantamount to ruling out anesthesia for surgery because patients have suffered permanent brain damage, or died, when an absent-minded anesthesiologist turned the wrong dial.

Try as they might, chelation critics have been unable to find more than a handful of patients harmed over the entire three decades. The vast majority of chelated patients who suffered adverse effects suffered during the 1960s, when chelation pioneers were still uncertain as to proper dose and administration of EDTA. Since then, chelation therapy has had a remarkable safety record.

Assuming, at worst, that over the years 25 patients have died of chelation out of the more than 400,000 treated. That is a mortality rate of less than one hundredth of one percent. Compare that to the death rate from bypass surgery—one to five percent.

Which brings us at last to the real danger of chelation—the one not even its advocates are publicly acknowledging. The real danger stems from the growing number of untrained, unqualified, unethical doctors jumping on the chelation bandwagon. Why now? Because every day chelation therapy is becoming better known and more sought after by growing numbers of people.

Recovered patients are outspoken salesmen. Even the tight-lipped are good advertisements—walking billboards. The more enthusiastic people become, and they have good reason for their enthusiasm, the more likelihood greedy opportunists will find ways to exploit the unwary. It is happening already.

The "quick-buck" boys are ready, waiting in the wings to cash in on the efforts of those who worked so hard and struggled for so many years to legitimize chelation and bring it to public attention.

Chelation "mills," for the most part laymen-owned, are springing up in many of the more populated areas of the country. They adhere to the supermarket concept of medical treatment, which holds the promise not of quality care for the patients, but financial gain for the operators.

Entrepreneur types, with aspirations of establishing nationwide networks, have already offered franchises to businessmen who can profit from chelation by hiring physicians to staff their premises, in some cases on a parttime, limited basis. Costs are often kept to a minimum by employing doctors untrained and inexperienced in chelation, or by using mainly paramedical personnel. They hire public relations firms to design high-power advertising campaigns to promote their clinics via overstated ads that are hypercritical of conventional medicine. They urge patients to elect chelation for anything and everything that might ail them.

In one such syndicate operation, the doctor hired to oversee and supervise patient care at three chelation clinics 60 miles apart was allegedly untrained in chelation other than a brief period spent observing treatment procedures. Investigation of his medical background revealed a questionable history. He had previously been involved with setting up large, profit-making "emergency" centers in a way that had so outraged the community that he had closed them overnight and allegedly skipped town, taking the investors' money with him and leaving huge debts.

In the first two weeks of its operation, this sham clinic was reported to have one cardiac arrest that we know of, but the patient was resuscitated. As of this writing, there have been no deaths, but legitimate chelationists are holding their breath. In place of the careful monitoring so vital to patient safety, patients are rushed through, with little or no individual attention, hooked up to IVs and turned loose. They are often given no nutritional supplementation, no diet, no instructions as to smoking, drinking, exercise, and the general lifestyle changes that are an integral part of complete chelation treatment.

Obviously, this situation must be addressed and controlled or chelation therapy will be destroyed just when universal acceptance is at hand. Chelation critics are quick to latch on to any excuse to feed disadvantageous tidbits to the sensation-hungry media.

Imagine their glee if Mike Wallace, Morley Safer, and the rest of the *Sixty Minutes* crew could zero in on a chelation center where 50 to 80 patients per day were "processed" without adequate medical supervision. Imagine the public outcry and repercussions triggered by an exposé documenting a chelation center where patients were chelated too rapidly (to effect a more profitable turnover) or too frequently, regardless of whether they have full kidney function, one kidney, half a kidney, or are close to kidney collapse.

There are such places. One of my patients, who had been previously chelated in another state, complained to me after her first treatment at my clinic, "Why did it take three hours, doctor? It went much faster where I was chelated before."

Despite well-established evidence that chelation infusions should be timed to last three hours or more, I have heard reports of 60-minute treatments. Chelation "supermarkets" are setting themselves up for the full *Sixty Minutes* treatment.

There are two real dangers at hand. The first is to the public at large—the danger of being treated by an incompetent or greedy chelator. The second is the possible end of chelation. There is no doubt chelation is in danger of being condemned because of the excesses of its exploiters. The same popularity that might soon make it possible for victims of cardiovascular disease to have easy access to a safe and effective nonsurgical procedure could doom that very therapy before it has the chance to save limbs and lives.

The professional association of physicians interested in promoting the competent and ethical use of chelation is attempting to weed out unqualified physicians. It has established the American Board of Chelation Therapy, which maintains standards of practice and certifies physicians only after they have taken training courses, have passed written and oral examinations, and have had supervised experience.

But this relatively small professional group cannot watch every aspect of the mushrooming chelation movement. For example, it cannot halt the aggressive marketing of so-called "oral chelators," being advertised to the public as capable of producing benefits similar to intravenous EDTA. Despite the glowing testimonials contained in ads for these nutritional substances, no oral chelator developed to date even comes close to being a suitable substitute. Potent chelating agents are too toxic to be routinely given orally. At one time EDTA was given by mouth, but the practice was quickly abandoned upon discovery that this increased the uptake of lead and also interfered with the proper absorption and utilization of essential nutritional elements.

AAMPS has neither the resources nor the clout to establish a fail-safe chelation environment. An informed patient is his own best protector. To avoid hazards, know what to look for and what questions to ask. Be wary of any physician that does not follow the recommended protocol described in this book which is the official accepted standard in use by the American Board of Chelation Therapy and the American Academy of Medical Preventics, and which, incidentally, was written personally by me.

11

The Chelation Experience

First timers have a pleasant surprise in store when they arrive for their initial chelation treatment. Even hospital phobics feel at home, reassured by the relaxed, informal, and friendly ambience characteristic of most treatment centers.

Unlike most forms of doctoring, being chelated is a group experience. Treatments are given in a comfortable, family-type room, furnished with cushioned easy chairs and recliners. You might think you had wandered into the lounge of a private club were not each of the dozen or more people who are napping, chatting, reading, or watching TV connected to a container of fluid dripping slowly into an arm or hand.

Newcomers respond well to the chatty, light-hearted atmosphere. Because patients spend long hours together, they are soon on a first-name basis, swapping medical experiences, diet tips, and snapshots of grandchildren. They talk politics, sports, exchange family histories, and, most important, provide encouragement and support for new patients.

You hear it so often.

"Don't worry. You'll do fine. Let me tell you the shape I was in when . . ."

What's it like to be chelated?

"It's like attending a family reunion, where you like all your relatives," a patient once remarked.

Others have said, "It's like my weekly visit to the beauty salon," or "like having group therapy," or, more to the point, "like joining a society where everyone shares a very special, common interest."

What's true of the Mount Rogers Clinic is also true of most other chelation facilities I have heard of or visited.

Ironically, chelation critics have tried to turn a plus—the pleasant surroundings and psychological support—into a minus. Many contend that patient recoveries can be attributed to the power of suggestion, as though chelationists were involved in some form of group hypnosis, bewitching patients into imagining themselves well.

Contradicting this oft-leveled charge is a report from an outstanding expert in veterinary medicine who happens to use EDTA chelation therapy on race horses. Dr. Lloyd S. McKibbon has observed remarkable changes in the racing performance of all treated animals, verified by physiological monitoring tests. If chelation is really only a placebo, as many opponents would have people believe, how amazing that even race horses can be fooled!

Indeed, were chelation specialists able to mesmerize people with blackened, gangrenous toes back to health with "think pink" suggestions, such feats, in themselves remarkable, would be worthy of acclaim on TV's *That's Incredible.*

I have no doubt that there are psychological benefits associated with chelation therapy. We do everything we can to encourage healing with lots of individual attention, group support, and hope.

Why such emphasis on the social environment?

Many chelation patients are very sick indeed, perhaps with a gangrenous extremity or at great risk of heart attacks or stroke. Not infrequently, they've been advised to face the inevitable by physicians who've told them nothing more could be done.

Our immediate goal is to reduce their anxiety. What better way then to expose them to firsthand testimonials. That's not the only reason we encourage conviviality. It makes life pleasant for everyone, staff and patients alike.

As a patient once told me, "I hate being around sick people. My best surprise was to find that no one acted sick. Even those patients I later discovered had really serious conditions were joking and smiling. In all my weeks of treatment, I don't remember anyone who looked really grim or sad. I certainly never saw anybody crying."

And a more practical lady remarked, "The worst part of being chelated is it's so boring. I'd go nuts if there weren't people to talk to."

Not that being chelated is all fun and games. It is, after all, a biochemically complex treatment. While it appears simple to the uninitiated, behind the scenes a highly sophisticated and carefully planned protocol regulates the course of individual treatments.

To give you a clearer understanding of the chelation experience, from both sides of the physician's desk, let's follow a mythical new patient step by step.

We'll call him Mr. B. He is 57, has had a well-documented heart attack (myocardial infarction), and he takes a full bottle of 100 nitroglycerin tablets each week, which only partially relieves his angina. He can't walk 100 yards with a small bag of groceries without stopping to catch his breath.

When he first called the office to inquire about chelation, Mr. B. was mailed an information packet.

On his first visit, he arrived prepared with a long list of questions typical of those most often asked about the procedure.

WHERE DO WE START?

With pretreatment testing. We start by obtaining a detailed medical history. We want to know all about you; not just your age, marital status, occupation, and all previous medical problems, but also about your family and their health status. You will be asked questions about your diet, your lifestyle, your good and bad habits, whether you drink or smoke, what doctor-prescribed or over-the-counter medications you take, how much you sleep, play, and exercise.

We will ask about symptoms—pains, headaches, dizzy spells, unusual fatigue, swelling of the hands or feet, palpitations, nervous spells, heart flutter, everything you can think of to fully answer the question, "How do you feel?" And we will arrange to get copies of pertinent past medical records from hospitals, doctors, or other available sources.

That's just for starters.

Next we do a complete hands-on, head-to-toe physical examination. We look in ears, eyes, nose, throat; we check for the regularity of pulses in neck, groin, and feet; then we listen to those same pulses with a stethoscope.

We check fingernails and earlobes for color, listen to breathing. We test for reflexes, examine the chest, listen to the heart, get blood pressure readings, and do some form of noninvasive vascular testing, such as the Doppler ultrasound, which measures blood flow adequacy in various parts of the body.

You'll be given an electrocardiogram and, if appropriate, a chest x-ray and possibly a stress test. Then a series of blood tests to ascertain the status of your biochemical health and determine whether you have diabetes, elevated cholesterol or other blood fats, abnormal carbohydrate metabolism, liver disease, kidney disease, anemia, infection, a compromised immune system, or other problems. You will be asked to collect a 24-hour urine specimen, which will be tested for creatinine clearance, a precise measure of kidney function. Finally, we'll snip off some hair to be sent off for analysis—the least expensive, easiest way to screen your nutritional mineral and trace element status and determine whether your body has accumulated excessive toxic metals.

WHEW! HOW LONG DOES ALL THAT TAKE?

Usually most of the day—anywhere from four to eight hours. It may then take another day or more to receive the complete results of biochemical tests.

WHAT'S NEXT?

Assuming the tests reveal your health status could be improved with a course of chelation treatments, and you have no contraindicating conditions, a treatment schedule will be recommended, to be adjusted periodically to your progress and individual tolerance.

I WANT TO KNOW EXACTLY WHAT TO EXPECT. WHAT IS THE PROCEDURE? HOW IS IT DONE? WHAT GOES IN THE BOTTLE? HOW WILL I FEEL?

After you are comfortably seated, a trained technician will begin your infusion. The prepared bottle of EDTA solution, hung at ceiling height on an adjustable stand, will be attached to a vein in the back of your hand or forearm via tubing ending in a tiny needle, which will be inserted as painlessly as possible. Most find the momentary pin prick a minimal discomfort. To keep the infusion set firmly in place, we tape the arm to a padded arm board, which then rests on a pillow. This provides greater comfort for the patient, and also allows him or her to move about more freely, without fear of dislocating the needle.

The technician will next adjust the drip rate as individually indicated. In most cases, it is timed to one drop per second for a three-plus-hour treatment. To make certain the infusion is being well tolerated, you will be carefully observed during the treatment session.

Prior to each treatment, we obtain both a urine and blood specimen to ensure that kidney function is adequate to excrete the EDTA infusion safely. If any evidence of overload is detected, or if there is a hint of kidney insufficiency, treatment is discontinued, or delayed, until the kidneys recover their normal reserve.

This continual checking procedure is especially important in elderly patients who commonly have reduced kidney function. Properly monitored, kidney overload can be avoided. In most cases, kidney function actually improves after a course of therapy.

As for the chelating solution, the infusion normally consists of 500 cc of intravenous solution containing EDTA, to which is added (according to individual needs) varying doses of vitamins and minerals. We generally add the B complex vitamins and Vitamin C, a weak chelating agent that enhances the ability of EDTA to remove lead and other toxic metals. Magnesium, beneficial for cardiovascular disease, is another common additive. We also include a bit of heparin, which is an anti-coagulant—not enough to thin the blood or prolong clotting time, but just enough to prevent a blood clot at the injection site. If you should experience any discomfort or pain during the infusion, we add a local anesthetic—procaine or lidocaine—the same substance your dentist uses. We don't want it to hurt, and it shouldn't.

Now, as to how you will feel. Everybody is different. Restless people, and those who are easily bored, should bring along something to busy themselves with: an entertaining book, study material, or a handiwork project, especially if they will not be content chatting, napping, or watching TV for three to four hours.

Patients must remain comparatively immobile while being treated. They can move about gingerly if they must: to go to the bathroom or take a telephone call, but for the most part it is best to stay in place to prevent disruption of the infusion.

The vast majority of patients consider each treatment a pleasant respite, especially if, as is quite common, they begin to feel beneficial effects after a few sessions. Once the treatments start to take hold, many people can breathe, walk, and work without discomfort after years of progressive deterioration, and they usually look forward to being chelated.

WHAT IF I HAVE TO INTERRUPT THE COURSE OF TREATMENT? OR MOVE AWAY? OR JUST DECIDE I WANT TO QUIT?

You can stop treatment anytime and still retain the benefits from all sessions up to that point. Benefits accrue in direct proportion to the number of treatments received. Unless you wait one year or longer between treatments, benefits start to add up again with each new treatment.

There is no rebound effect with chelation, nor worsening of symptoms merely because treatments are stopped. Once you start, you do not have to be chelated periodically unless you want to.

You can start treatment with one doctor and continue with another in some other part of the country, usually with no difficulty. The treatment protocol might vary a bit, but it should not be significantly different.

AND WHAT ABOUT SIDE EFFECTS?

While once in a while someone encounters a minor medical problem during chelation, chances are you won't. Among the possible side effects are the following:

- The EDTA infusion might cause minor irritation—a burning or stinging, or some slight swelling, or a black and blue mark at the puncture site.
- An occasional patient develops a skin rash, either as an allergic reaction or related to the body's loss of certain vitamins, such as B_6, and elements such as zinc, even though these substances are supplemented during treatment. When necessary, we add more.
- The therapy may upset your stomach, even make you feel nauseated, a problem readily treated with medicine or more vitamin B_6. This adverse effect is experienced by less than one percent of all patients.
- An occasional patient develops a headache. If so, simple pain medication relieves it.

- Once in a great while, a patient experiences sudden feelings of faintness, weakness, light-headedness, extreme fatigue, or dizziness if he stands up suddenly during or after treatment. This may be because blood pressure can become a bit lower during treatment. In fact, many with high blood pressure have their anti-hypertension medication dosages decreased after chelation therapy. The immediate solution is to rest for an extra hour or so after treatment, with feet elevated, head lowered, until blood pressure has normalized.
- If you are hypoglycemic, you may experience a weak feeling or feel a bit "whoozy" during chelation because blood sugar levels may drop. A glass of fruit juice, or better yet a meal before treatment, will minimize the hypoglycemic reaction.
- One out of an estimated 5000 patients develop an unexplained fever within the first 24 hours after chelation. It usually disappears spontaneously without treatment, but should be brought to the physician's attention.
- Approximately one in 20 patients develop leg cramps, usually at night. EDTA does effect calcium-magnesium balances, and additional magnesium in the intravenous solution markedly ameliorates this problem.
- One percent of patients develop a loose stool or diarrhea either immediately after treatment or the next day. This is remedied by anti-diarrhea medication. More common is the need to empty the bladder more frequently. Some people report they have to get up once or twice at night. EDTA is a mild diuretic. Therapy improves tissue integrity, decreasing soft tissue edema, returning accumulated fluids to the circulatory system to be excreted. That's why many patients experience an unexpected reward—a three- to five-pound weight loss.
- Diabetic patients must have their blood sugar carefully monitored to prevent inadvertent hyperinsulism. Patients who use insulin will usually notice that blood sugar is easier to control and that insulin doses can be gradually reduced, and occasionally eliminated, during and after a course of chelation therapy.

HOW MANY TREATMENTS? OVER HOW LONG A PERIOD OF TIME?

We won't have the answer to those questions until the results of your medical exams are in, and even then we can only estimate from experience. It's a highly individualized matter. Individuals being chelated preventively, prior to the onset of disease symptoms, normally require fewer treatments: 20 to begin with, and then five to ten a year thereafter for maximum benefits. In cases where there is an established history of angina attacks, or other signs of arterial disease, we usually prescribe a series of 30 treatments over a three to five-month period, after which we recommend one follow-up treatment every two weeks, or as needed to maintain improvement

CAN YOU GUARANTEE RESULTS?

Of course not, even though chelation has an enviable record. While better than 75 percent of all patients treated experience a reduction of symptoms related to arteriosclerotic-type ailments, it is no panacea for all the health problems that accompany the aging process. It does not "cure" old age. Sooner or later, human mortality catches up with us, chelated or not.

Chelation delays the inevitable. It helps most people live longer and healthier, but only to the extent that they are willing to modify their lifestyles.

For example, patients *must* quit smoking. Those who continue to use tobacco in any form jeopardize their chance of benefit. I often tell my patients that to continue to use tobacco while undergoing chelation is analagous to pouring kerosene on a fire while calling for the fire department to put it out. Failure to follow an active exercise program, as prescribed, may also decrease potential benefits. It is equally important for patients to adhere as closely as possible to recommended nutritional guidelines.

HOW WILL I KNOW CHELATION IS WORKING?

Seriously ill patients, those with advanced forms of atherosclerotic-related ailments, rarely have reason to ask that question. Day by day, they enjoy an improved ability to function in a more normal way. A typical illustration is Mr. D., who, prior to chelation, could barely make his way from living room couch to dining room table. Six months after treatments began, he retiled his roof, and did the work single-handedly in below freezing temperature.

Patients who are chelated preventively will see more subtle indications. Complexions take on a more youthful glow, partly because of improved circulation and partly because of a gradual reduction in the skin wrinkling resulting from cross-linkage damage due to excess free radical activity. Hair condition—color and texture—often improves. That is because increased levels of internally produced anti-oxidants and fewer free radicals sometimes help to stop hair loss and dandruff, and occasionally cause gray or white hair to return to its original color.

One more proof that chelation is doing its job: those telltale brown spots (aptly called age spots) begin to fade away. The same free radical reactions that cause deterioration to skin, tissues, and organs throughout the body give rise to yellow-brown frecklelike marks (most noticeable on hands). These are visible evidence that cellular wastes are building up in your entire physiological system. Over a period of several months, chelation speeds the removal of these cellular wastes, and the ugly age spots gradually disappear, a far better solution to the problem than widely advertised commercial "fade-liver-spots creams" designed to "bleach" the skin clear.

I'VE RUN OUT OF QUESTIONS.

Let me answer the one important question you failed to ask: How can you be assured of a chelating physician's competence?

As with many other medical procedures, you should investigate the knowledge, experience, and credentials of the physician you select.

To protect yourself, ask if the doctor you are considering is certified in chelation as a diplomate of the American Board of Chelation Therapy (ABCT). If he is, you can be assured he has at least passed minimal requirements, including written and oral tests, and has been supervised treating patients.

If there is no ABCT-certified physician convenient, make certain that the chelating physician you are consulting has completed sufficient course work to pass the ABCT's written exam. Don't be bashful. Ask, and above all, don't sign a treatment consent form unless you're convinced you're in safe hands.

To protect yourself against being victimized by a "chelation mill," watch for these telltale omissions:

- Failure to obtain a complete medical history, including previous hospital records, recent x-ray reports, EKGs, arteriograms, or other lab tests.
- Failure to do a thorough hands-on physical examination, if not done and recorded recently elsewhere. This should include a

one-on-one inquiry into such lifestyle habits as eating, smoking, exercise, and drinking, a comprehensive series of blood tests, a 24-hour urine collection, and some form of noninvasive vascular testing.

Once chelation treatments have begun, there are other warning signs to watch out for:

- Failure of the physician or his staff to collect urine and blood samples prior to each chelation treatment, or to periodically (once every ten treatments) request 24-hour urine collections.
- Failure of the physician or office personnel, when asked, to supply information about tests, or answer questions about procedures, symptoms, or progress.
- Failure to receive personalized, individual attention. One- to two-hour chelation rush-through infusions are the hallmark of "chelation mills."

No treatment is any better than the physician administering it. Unfortunately, there are quack chelationists around, just as there are opportunists in every other medical specialty.

One chelation doctor I heard of claimed to be using a patented secret formula not available to other doctors, for which he charged two to three times the going EDTA chelation fee. Subsequent analysis revealed he was using the same EDTA as everyone else.

Your best protection is to be an informed patient. When your doctor balks at answering questions, it might be time to seek another physician.

12

Bye-Bye Bypass

In the two centuries that have passed since the classical description of angina pectoris first appeared in medical literature, there has been little for physicians to offer patients in the way of effective treatment until comparatively recently.

Right through the end of the 1940s, nitroglycerin was the standard treatment for pain relief. At the onset of an angina episode, a victim placed a tiny white pill under the tongue and waited for the uncomfortably tight, strangling sensation and pains to subside. But because the condition underlying angina is usually progressive, pains became more frequent and severe, and less amenable to nitroglycerin relief.

The seriously afflicted had little choice but to learn to live with their condition. Since exertion predictably triggered frightening discomfort, many were forced to adopt curtailed lifestyles, giving up former work and play activities.

In 1950, a seemingly miraculous remedy captured attention. Surgeons developed a new operation called internal mammary artery ligation, which involved surgical tying off the mammary artery, which carries blood to the chest region. Because this artery is near the heart, surgeons hoped this action would force blood to flow through other arteries (including coronary arteries) in the vicinity and ease the pain of angina.

Results exceeded the most optimistic expectations. Remarkably, up to 90 percent of patients reported either total pain relief or dramatic symptom improvement. The operation, hailed as a miraculous advance, was widely advocated by many members of the medical profession. Enthusiasm mounted; angina victims lined up; surgeons maintained three-month waiting lists. The operation's effectiveness went unquestioned, and untested, for almost ten years.

But then, as now, there were skeptics within the medical community. There was too much enthusiasm to suit some analytic physicians, who doubted the procedure deserved such universal acclaim inasmuch as it had no scientific rationale. The doubters arranged to verify the surgery's effectiveness with a research protocol unacceptable under today's more rigid ethical standards.

They set out to test the procedure by dividing surgical candidates into two groups, each equally afflicted with angina. All subjects were told they were to undergo ligation surgery, and went through identical hospital protocols with only one important difference: One group did have the ligation operation while the control group was taken into the operating room, anesthetized, and then subjected to a sham operation. Their chests were opened, then closed. When they awoke, they were told their operations had been successful.

To the astonishment of the entire medical community, the surgeons included, both groups reported relief from anginal pain and increased tolerance of exercise, but the group that had undergone the sham surgery fared better than those who had undergone the genuine operation. It was the first time medical researchers proved the placebo effect extends to surgery, and, not surprisingly, when word got out, the number of operations plummeted.

What has this to do with current methods of treating angina?

More than one leading scientist has expressed the belief that coronary bypass surgery, the most common major operation performed in the United States today, is the 1980s equivalent of the sham surgery of the 1950s. Said one, "My own suspicion is that a placebo might do just as well, and not cost $50 thousand, the usual price tag of a coronary bypass operation."

Despite the hoopla surrounding the bypass procedure, it has never been conclusively proven to do anything but relieve the pain of angina. As with any symptom-relieving treatment, there is a real possibility that the placebo effect is at least in part responsible.

The bypass procedure may also serve as a type of "surgical beta-blocker," with an action paralleling that of a group of drugs that diminish pain by interfering with nerve impulses that trigger arterial spasm and heart muscle contraction and bring on angina. It is not widely known, but it is impossible to perform the operation without partially disrupting the nerves that stimulate the beta receptors on arteries and heart muscle.

Is bypass surgery, like the operation that preceded it by some 20 years, undeservedly popular?

When the Office of Technical Assessment was commissioned by the U.S. Congress to review the case for surgery for coronary artery disease, it was not favorably impressed. The panel of government consultants, which included leading academicians from the nation's most prestigious medical schools, reached its conclusions in 1978 and reported:

"For more than half a century, surgeons have believed that an efficacious surgical approach to coronary artery disease is possible. Prior to the modern bypass operation, five different operations were developed and advocated enthusiastically. Although all five operations were ultimately abandoned as of no value, initially they were alleged to be efficacious, with reports in the medical literature claiming 'objective' evidence of benefits."

Noting that "coronary bypass surgery seems to give excellent symptomatic relief from angina pectoris . . . but the improvement diminishes with time," they cautioned there was a historical lesson to be heeded, pointing out "the possible placebo effect (of bypass surgery) needs to be kept in mind because: (1) the initial results are similar to previous operations; (2) nonsurgical treatment also produces good results; and (3) the methods of evaluation of symptomatic relief are experiential."

The chief of cardiology at the Montreal Heart Institute, Dr. Lucien Campeau, is yet another cardiovascular specialist who suspects long-term relief of angina pain results from what he calls a "pain-denial placebo effect." Dr. Campeau came to this conclusion after studying 235 patients angiographically three years after their coronary artery bypass operations, discovering that even in those cases where grafts had reclosed, patients unexpectedly reported being improved or angina-free.

An August 1983 article in the *Journal of the American Medical Association* once again documented angina pain relief in 75 percent of patients who have bypass surgery. Shortly thereafter, an article in the *New England Journal of Medicine* stated 75 percent of angina patients' pain is relieved no matter what you do. In effect, these two highly authoritative articles are saying bypass surgery works just about as good as a placebo.

Many patients who opt for this operation have a real need to believe in its effectiveness. They have a huge emotional investment in a successful outcome, often having been scared into believing that this surgery is the only way to save their lives.

Claims that the operation prolongs life are still being debated. When the Harvard University School of Public Health put coronary bypass surgery to the test, they concluded it is often unnecessary. The Harvard study involved 142 men who had all "flunked" a treadmill exercise test, and had evidenced other indications of extensive coronary atherosclerosis. Each had been advised to undergo the bypass operation.

But when this group of surgical candidates was referred to Harvard specialists for a second opinion, surgery was rejected in favor of a drug, diet, and exercise program. After keeping tabs on these 142 men for anywhere from 20 months to 12 years, the Harvard researchers found their death rate exactly what would have been expected had the men been operated on (provided, the study pointed out, they survived the operation, which has an operative mortality of two to three percent).

Contrary to the claims of cardiovascular surgeons, bypass surgery does nothing to improve the outlook for survival, according to the Harvard report.

A study by Dr. Wilbert Aranow of the University of California at Irvine that compared atherosclerotic patients treated surgically with those treated medically also revealed no evidence of increased survival or lowered heart attack risk. Nor did studies conducted by Duke University Medical Center find reason to suggest that coronary surgery prolongs life in comparison with medical management.

An analysis of 1101 consecutive patients with coronary artery disease—490 had surgery, 611 were treated medically—was made by the Division of Cardiology and Department of Community Health Sciences. At the end of four years, there was no significant difference in the survival rate between the surgically treated and the medically treated: 82 percent for the first group; 78 percent for the second.

When the Federal government's long-awaited ten-year study of bypass surgical outcomes was released, it offered little encouragement for advocates of cardiovascular surgery. The study was conducted at 11 prominent medical centers: the University of Alabama, Alabama Medical College, Boston University, the Marshfield (Wis.) Clinic, Massachusetts General Hospital, Milwaukee Veterans Hospital, New York University, St. Louis University, Stanford University, Yale University, and at the Montreal Heart Institute. It collected data on 780 volunteer patients with mild heart disease or heart symptoms, divided into two groups. Ninety percent of the patients were men. Their average age was 51, and none was over 65. Half had bypass operations; the other half had medical treatment consisting of drugs and advice to start exercising sensibly and avoid risks like smoking, overeating, and consuming too much fat in their diets.

After six years, 92 percent of the surgical patients and 90 percent of the medical patients are still alive. The researchers concluded that an estimated 25,000 bypass operations could be eliminated each year. That is fine as far as it goes. But the real question to be asked is, did the scientists speak out boldly enough?

Many think not. There is good reason to suspect they were extremely conservative in their estimate of the annual number of unneeded operations and downplayed their statements concerning the percentage of bypasses that could safely be avoided.

As Dr. Eugene Braunwald, professor of cardiology at Harvard Medical School, pointed out in the *New England Journal of Medicine*, the data was already obsolete when the study came out, inasmuch as it was collected before the advent of newer medical therapies such as calcium blockers and improved beta-blockers.

"Nonsurgical therapy has not stood still during the last six years," Dr. Braunwald noted, challenging the validity of findings that exclude recent advances in nonsurgical cardiovascular treatment.

Were the researchers too kind to proponents of surgery? If bypass surgery is probably no better than less drastic treatments, does it do any harm?

A U.S. government pamphlet entitled "Medicine for the Layman—Heart Attacks," published by the Department of Health, Education and Welfare, noted clinical investigations have yet to determine whether bypass surgery improves or impairs heart function. As stated by this booklet, "There is no evidence yet that bypass surgery makes the heart pump better—some evidence bypass surgery may actually decrease efficiency."

One risk of surgery is the real possibility of suffering a heart attack while still on the operating table. Reports suggest that happens to upwards of five percent of all patients and 40 percent of some high-risk patients. In very rare instances, the heart may refuse to resume beating when taken off bypass.

Neurological damage can be another distressing aftermath of surgery. Few researchers have investigated the frequency or severity of post-bypass neurological complications, but a 1980 study reported about two percent of the 421 patients studied suffered central nervous system damage severe enough to affect functioning: paralysis, inability to speak, and blindness. A larger percentage suffered transitory neurological problems such as confusion, memory loss, weakness, tingling in hands, arms, or legs, and numbness. Most, but not all, of those problems gradually disappeared with time.

Not to be overlooked is the psychological trauma. It would be difficult to find anyone who is not terrorized by the operation. Bypass patients must also face the possibility that one operation won't do it. Reports indicate 15 to 30 percent of vein grafts become occluded within one year of surgery, and there is some evidence that the operation itself accelerates atherosclerosis in the graft-receptor arteries.

The ultimate damage—death.

While few deny the bypass operation involves serious hazards, there is enormous disagreement on mortality rates, reported at anywhere from 1 to 42 percent, depending on where the procedure is done, who performs the surgery, on which group of patients, and on how data is collected. The National Heart and Lung Institute has reported the risk of death following coronary artery bypass surgery to be between one and four percent in the best of circumstances and 10 to 15 percent in the worst.

Surgical candidates are understandably quoted the most optimistic view, even though their chances of survival depend to a large degree on their age, general health status, degree of disease, and the skill and experience of the surgeon and surgical team.

The testing procedures upon which surgical decisions are based are also open to criticism. Each new diagnostic device that comes along gets tacked on the ever-growing check list. Physicians may become so captivated with space-age diagnostics that they fail to remember they're treating patients, not tests. Coronary arteriograms, electrocardiograms, radionuclide studies, nuclear ventriculograms, thallium scans, digital subtraction arteriography, ultrasound imaging, treadmill stress tests, and echocardiography are all occasionally useful, but overused, according to no less an authority than Dr. George Burch, professor of cardiology at Tulane University School of Medicine.

As Dr. Burch points out, "It has yet to be demonstrated that the new information, expensively gotten, will change the way we treat patients."

What he failed to mention is how often such diagnostic procedures merely serve as an excuse to speed a patient into surgery.

The Harvard University study, previously mentioned, specifically challenged the over-reliance of many heart specialists on exercise tests. The researchers noted that stress tests suggesting clogged arteries are an insufficient basis by themselves for the decision to undertake such procedures as coronary angiography as a prelude to surgery, the common current practice.

Exercise stress tests are not only inconclusive, but also carry some small risk. A study of 170,000 such tests revealed that for every 10,000 persons tested, one may die and two or three may require hospitalization. Occasionally, emergency treatment is needed. While the risk of death is relatively low, 0.01 to 0.04 percent, that still seems excessively high considering, in many cases, the test results may be vague or misleading.

For almost 30 years, the coronary angiogram has been the diagnostic tool most revered by vascular surgeons, the one they invariably rely on for evidence for the need for surgery.

In principle, the angiogram (also called an arteriogram) provides a filmed visualization of dye injected into the arteries, enabling skilled radiologists to pinpoint the location and precise (expressed in percentages) extent of blockages. Radiological readings are rarely challenged. If the angiographer reports as much as a 75 percent occlusion of the so-called "time-bomb artery" (the left main anterior descending artery), the necessity for a bypass is considered confirmed.

Have patients gone to surgery on the basis of misinterpreted arteriograms?

"Without question," according to Dr. Arthur Selzer, cardiopulmonary lab chief at San Francisco's Presbyterian Hospital, who told a reporter he had "always been skeptical about angiographic readings, especially when expressed in percentages. That implies the evaluator is measuring something when he's just giving a visual impression of an obstruction."

It was not until the National Heart, Lung and Blood Institute (NHLBI) undertook an investigation of angiogram reliability that cardiologists were given hard evidence that coronary angiography is more art than science.

The NHLBI report, presented at the 1979 American Heart Association meeting in Anaheim, California, revealed that inaccurate assessments of arteriograms are commonplace and that when experienced radiologists evaluate the same angiograms, they have conflicting opinions almost half the time.

The NHLBI conducted a three-pronged probe. In one study, three arteriographers, working independently, examined films of 28 patients who had died within 40 days of cardiac catheterization. When their readings of the amount of occlusion of that all-important left main artery were compared with actual postmortem findings, it turned out they were more often wrong than right. In a whopping 82 percent of their judgments, the degree of narrowing was significantly under- or overestimated.

In the second stage of the research project, 30 films with distinct pathology were circulated among radiologists at three first-rate medical centers to discover how often first, second, and third opinions might agree. The discouraging results: only 61 percent of the time did two or more of the three groups reach the same conclusion.

Finally, in the third study, three months later, the same 30 films were recirculated to the same experienced radiologists, who did not know, of course, they were being asked to reevaluate films they had seen before. This time, the radiologists not only disagreed with each other, they also disagreed with themselves! In 32 percent of the readings, their second evaluations differed from their first.

Exploding the myth of angiogram reliability had "profound implications for the diagnosis and treatment of coronary disease," declared Dr. Harvey G. Kemp, Jr., cardiology chief at St. Luke's Medical Center in New York, who had directed one segment of the research. Especially, he noted, since the evaluations had been conducted under the most favorable circumstances. "We had some of the best people reading the best quality angiograms available," he pointed out.

And how did the cardiovascular community respond to research that clearly indicated patients were being scheduled for surgery based on erroneous diagnoses? They didn't. Nothing's changed.

Despite findings to the contrary, the coronary angiogram remains the "gold standard" of cardiovascular diagnosis and is still considered the final word when it comes to determining if bypass surgery is indicated. In 1982, an estimated 400,000 angiograms were performed nationwide.

To refer to the angiogram, which costs about $2500 (almost as much as a full course of chelation) and usually requires a one- to-five-day hospitalization, as a diagnostic test, is in itself misleading when, in fact, it is an operation to get the patient ready for an operation. The recommendation for surgery is often a foregone conclusion.

Occluded arteries are to be expected. Remember, atherosclerotic plaque begins accumulating before the third decade of life, and many men and women who are symptom-free and considered healthy have been found to have 75 percent or more arterial blockage when autopsied after accidental death from causes unrelated to arterial disease.

Of all the diagnostic procedures, the angiogram is the one patients fear most—"Worse than the surgery which followed," many report. It can be a long, uncomfortable procedure, involving catherization through an artery in the arm or groin, which is guided up into the heart. Dye is then injected through the catheter directly into the patient's coronary arteries. X-ray films of the dye flow through blood vessels ostensibly show the location, pattern, and extent of blockages, but as we've already learned, error-ridden readings of those films degrade their diagnostic value.

The best reason not to employ angiography as a routine testing tool is that it is relatively hazardous. Death rates from the procedure vary from 0.1 to 1.0 percent. It can also trigger a heart attack or stroke, either immediately or several months later, result in torn arteries, infection, or allergic reaction to the dye.

Finally, angiograms too often lead to a hazardous operation. Once the cardiologist requests an angiogram, the patient is frequently on the final lap of the surgical track.

If bypass surgery is an expensive, high-risk, limited benefit procedure, as research indicates, why then does it continue to be the uncontested winner of the "Most Popular Operation of the Year" award? Why do approximately 200,000 Americans a year now submit to a surgical procedure costing between $20,000 and $50,000 which will not cure their underlying disease and has a slight chance of making them worse? Good question.

Bypass surgery, a dramatic operation with lots of pizzazz, has been the beneficiary of considerable media "hype." In the early 1970s, it represented the ultimate in sophisticated medical technology, made possible by newly perfected heart-lung bypass machinery. Newspapers, magazines, and TV, always eager to publicize science with "soap opera" appeal, zoomed in to capture every heart-throbbing moment of what was hailed as a medical marvel.

The general public responded as might be expected. People with angina and other heart-related problems began seeking out cardiac surgeons, sometimes without even consulting their family physician. The medical community reacted just as naively. It's not just the average man in the street who learns what's new in medicine from the *National Enquirer*; surveys have shown many doctors also rely on lay publications to stay current on medical issues. Unperturbed by the lack of proven advantages over other therapies, cardiovascular physicians embraced the new technology with questionable enthusiasm.

Almost overnight, bypass surgery became a medical fad. An experimental procedure when first introduced, it has since become the treatment of choice for 165,000 or more Americans each year. Indeed, in certain social circles, the sternum splitting scar is a status symbol.

"What, you haven't had your bypass yet?" one executive asks another. The intimation is clear: only an administrator unworthy of having a key to the executive bathroom would have escaped the inevitable consequences of being dedicated to one's job. More recently, the question has changed somewhat, from, "Have you had your bypass?" to "How many arteries?" In several large metropolitan cities, being scheduled for cardiovascular surgery opens the door to the local "Zipper Club."

A prestigious procedure? Of course. It has a glamorous image since so many really important, famous people have had it—former Secretaries of State Henry Kissinger and Alexander Haig, King Khalid of Saudi Arabia, actor Rock Hudson, comedian Danny Kaye, top country music singer Marty Robbins. This two-time Grammy winner, by the way, had two bypasses: first a triple-bypass in 1970; then an 8-hour quadruple bypass in December of 1982. He died one week after the second operation.

The latest wrinkle among the elite is to have bypass surgery preventively. I'm not sure what that means, but when the 49-year-old governor of Kentucky, John Y. Brown, Jr., suffered chest pains while barbecuing the family's dinner, he was rushed to King's Daughters Hospital and 24 hours later underwent a triple bypass. His doctors told the press the operation was "preventive," emphasizing the governor had not had a heart attack, giving the totally unfounded impression the surgery would ward one off.

All of which serves to prove the rich, successful, and famous often get no better medical advice than the less privileged.

Would coronary bypass surgery have proliferated so rapidly and enjoyed such unwarranted popularity if it weren't so enormously profitable? Many critics believe it is a procedure that has gotten out of hand primarily because of the big bucks involved.

"Every time a surgeon does a heart bypass, he takes home a new sports car," quipped one cynic, referring to the $15,000 or more price tag that has provided some cardiovascular surgeons with incomes of $1 million per year, and more.

Nor are surgeons the only beneficiaries. Coronary artery bypass surgery is now an estimated $3.3 billion a year industry, providing a financial windfall to hospitals, drug and equipment manufacturers, and guaranteed employment to a small army of highly specialized, highly paid surgical and post-surgical coronary care teams. Economists forecast that if present growth rate continues, by 1986 bypass surgery will become a $7 billion business.

With third-party insurers picking up a large part of the tab, "some nonsurgical measures may be getting overlooked in the rush to get cases in the operating room," according to the executive director of Maryland's Health Services Cost Review Commission. "Less expensive treatments would get greater play if patients were uninsured and had to form 'first' opinions about their own money, instead of spending someone elses," he added.

Will criticism from within or without the medical community stem the flood to the surgical suites?

"Not likely," said one of San Francisco's leading cardiologists. "There's too much money involved. It's become a self-perpetuating industry."

Perhaps the surgeons have gotten carried away, but that's no reason for patients to play along.

Should you be advised to submit to bypass surgery before other treatments are fairly tried, ask this question first: "What are my other alternatives?"

13

You Have Other Alternatives

What are the alternatives to bypass surgery? The day it could be crucial for you to know, you might not have time to find out.

Consider what happened to 48-year-old Richard J., an advertising agency executive, when he, like a million and half other American men and women each year, had a heart attack without warning.

Richard had just finished lunch with a client and was heading back to the office when the terrible chest pains struck. Overweight, overstressed, underactive, a two-martini lunch man and a smoker, Richard suspected the worst as the ambulance rushed him to the hospital.

When Alice J. arrived, doctors were ready with a diagnosis—advanced atherosclerosis with three-vessel disease—and a remedy—immediate bypass surgery.

The cardiologist tried to be reassuring.

"Your husband's a lucky man," he said. "He's had a heart attack, and is under sedation, but he's doing okay. We've located his trouble. These films show the arteries that are blocked."

"What now?"

"We've scheduled surgery for first thing tomorrow, but he's in no condition to okay the operating permit. Sign here."

Mrs. J. vaguely recalled reading something about bypass surgery, but could not remember whether it was good or bad. She thought of Dick's friends, his golf buddy who'd died on the operating table and the art director who'd had his bypass five years ago and who looked and felt better than ever before.

"Right away?"

"There's no time to fool around," cautioned the surgeon. "Your husband's a walking time bomb. He could live forever, or die any minute. Those clogged arteries are keeping oxygen from reaching his heart."

What would you do? Would you stand your ground and insist on more time? Would you swallow your doubts and hope for the best?

Given all the facts and an opportunity to weigh the comparative risks and benefits of surgery and other modern nonsurgical treatment programs, I have no doubt most people would bypass the bypass.

But they are not often given the chance. In one instance, the surviving family of a man who had died during a bypass operation struck back. They instituted a class-action lawsuit against the university hospital, alleging the heart surgery booklet they had been given concealed the hospital's excessively high mortality rates, thus negating the validity of the operating permit because it was not signed with "informed" consent. In a similar case, the family sued because they were told about chelation after their dad died during bypass surgery.

Is a physician bound to inform you of all alternatives, those he disapproves of as well as those he endorses? Ethically, yes. Legally, not always.

Some doctors think modern medicine is too complicated to discuss with the average person.

Some doctors are so steeped in the jargon of their medical mystique that they are unable to describe things in understandable, simple English.

Some doctors appropriate the decision-making responsibility, assuming patients and their families, traumatized by a medical urgency, are too confused to think for themselves.

Some doctors are so prejudiced in favor of their own specialty that they disregard the benefits of competitive therapies.

Some doctors have simply failed to keep up with medical advances and new research.

And, let's face it, some doctors have too much invested in their specialized skills to be interested in therapies requiring retraining.

Nevertheless, in the last 15 years, medicine has taken some giant steps toward the conquest of heart disease. No better way to document progress than to realize some 200,000 Americans living today would have died during 1982 were it not for scientific breakthroughs on many fronts—from prevention to cure. Doctors know more about helping people get well; people know more about keeping themselves healthy.

To maintain control over your life, even when faced with a serious health reversal, do not give up your decision-making perogatives. Ask questions, be well read, keep an open mind, and inform yourself.

What are your alternatives if you reject bypass surgery? You have already learned a great deal about chelation therapy; now let's look at other possibilities, as well.

DRUGS. Long-term therapy with prescription drugs can be helpful when the basic health problem is an impairment of coronary artery blood flow, angina, arrhythmia, hypertension, or other conditions symptomatic of atherosclerosis and heart disease.

Drugs that might be recommended include the following:

Anti-coagulants: Primarily useful in diseases of the veins, such as thrombophlebitis, where there is a danger of blood clots forming and breaking loose.

Anti-coagulants are blood thinners and must be carefully used lest they precipitate hemorrhage. This is clearly a potential hazard, since the most common of these drugs is warfarin, found in hardware stores, where it's sold as rat poison. When rats eat enough, they bleed to death.

Anti-coagulants are rarely appropriate for patients with angina or atherosclerotic disease unless the danger of a blood clot embolizing from the wall of the heart is greater than the danger of possible hemorrhage as a result of the therapy. If your physician recommends such drugs, you might want a second opinion.

A less hazardous approach to decreasing the likelihood of blood clots, but with only slight benefit, involves aspirin or persantin, both thought to help decrease platelet "stickiness." There is some new evidence that small daily doses of aspirin may reduce the risk of heart attacks and strokes.

Another approach to this same problem is through a change in diet (to be described in a later chapter). But heed this warning:

> ***Do not go on the anti-free radical diet or make any changes in your food habits or take aspirin or any other new medicine without consulting your doctor if you are currently taking anti-coagulants. If you do, what may have been a safe dose may become a fatal dose.***

Blood vessel dilators: That old standby nitroglycerin is still used, and still appropriate, for relief of angina. It, like more recently developed short- or long-acting nitrates, such as Isordil, reduces spasm in blood vessels and decreases the workload of the heart. Angina is often relieved when the heart does not have to pump so hard. While drugs in this category do nothing to treat the underlying disease, they may in some cases reduce the risk of heart attack by reducing spasm strain on the heart.

New forms of this old drug include Transderm-Nitro (and similar products), adhesive patches impregnated with nitroglycerin, and a nitroglycerin skin ointment. Slow-release nitrates may be useful prior to exertion such as lovemaking or tennis.

While the nitrates can be very effective, either as a stopgap measure or for long-term use, they have their dark side. Among the more commonly observed adverse reactions are severe and persistent headaches, transient episodes of dizziness and weakness, and occasional skin rashes. If their use is interrupted, without a gradual tapering off, angina or even a heart attack may be precipitated.

Beta-blockers: Now marketed under dozens of trade names (Inderal, Blocadren, Tenormin, Lopressor), these drugs work on the body's adrenergic nervous system, which is involved in stimulating the activity of the heart and blood vessels in stressful situations. They interfere with the transmission of nerve impulses that trigger beta receptors, allowing relaxation of arteries and reducing the heart's oxygen requirements.

There is now substantial evidence that beta-blockers reduce the incidence—and severity—of first heart attacks and reduce the risk of death from recurrent heart attacks.

Variations of prototype beta-blockers more recently synthesized are expanding their usefulness. Used either alone or in conjunction with other medicines, they effectively control both angina and hypertension.

A substantial percentage of patients experience a variety of unpleasant side effects (not as often with the newer beta-blockers): sleeplessness, bad dreams, lowered sex drive, reduced energy. As one patient put it: "My get up and go, just got up and went."

Beta-blockers can present problems for asthmatics and people with respiratory problems by constricting the bronchioles in the lungs.

Calcium channel blockers: By interfering with the flow of calcium into heart and arterial muscle cells, calcium blockers reduce the intensity of the heart's contraction, and may interrupt or eliminate arrhythmias. They also allow the heart to rest more and reduce its need for oxygen. At the same time, they reduce spasm in the coronary arteries, increasing the blood flow and oxygen supply to the heart.

Also called calcium antagonists, these drugs have been used successfully in almost 60 countries for more than a decade. European doctors have found them amazingly helpful in reducing angina, treating heart rhythm disturbances, relieving hypertension, and preventing heart attacks.

A powerful group of drugs, they seem to be safer than many other medications, with few negative effects in most patients. Some calcium blockers are proving as effective as beta-blockers in the treatment of hypertension, with the advantage that they do not affect the lungs.

With the ability to reduce the damage that occurs when calcium leaks into cells where it does not belong, calcium blockers duplicate just one of the many therapeutic actions of chelation.

Cholesterol-lowering or lipid-lowering substances: Medications in this category, much like low-cholesterol diets, put the cart before the horse inasmuch as they are aimed at attacking the symptom rather than the problem. Drugs that lower blood cholesterol levels have not been shown to reduce the risk of heart attack. All cause nasty side effects, including impairment of liver function and an increased risk of gallstones and cancer. They may be indicated for patients with a hereditary tendency to very high blood cholesterol.

Digitalis: Under certain conditions, digitalis may relieve heart arrhythmias. Under other conditions, digitalis may produce heart arrhythmias. In certain patients, digitalis may relieve angina. There is an equal possibility that it can aggravate angina.

The role of digitalis in treating coronary heart disease is very speculative (it may relieve symptoms of heart failure); it should not be used routinely. If your doctor prescribes it, you may want a second opinion. The toxic dose of digitalis is so close to the effective therapeutic dose that potential benefits must be substantial to offset the risk.

Clot-dissolving enzymes: Streptokinase, a material produced by strep bacteria in a culture medium and then purified, is a clot-dissolving chemical which, when injected, can either stop a heart attack in progress or eliminate existing clots in veins or arteries. Urokinase, a similar agent, comes from human kidney cells grown in culture. Neither dissolves clots directly, but each stimulates the body's own clot-dissolving capabilities, restoring circulation. They also reduce platelet stickiness and probably help relax arterial spasm as well.

To effectively stop a heart attack, clot-dissolving enzymes must be used promptly. The patient must be in the right place—the hospital—at the right time—that is, with a trained physician standing by. In most cases, catheterization is necessary to locate the site of the clot.

Treatments with streptokinase or urokinase can be extremely valuable in heart attack emergencies, but have no impact on the atherosclerotic process involved in clot formation.

Every drug, misused, can be dangerous. Protect yourself. Seek the care of a skilled physician. Adhere to these do's and don'ts of proper drug-taking:

- DON'T stop taking drugs just because you are feeling better. Consult your doctor even if you no longer experience the symptoms for which the drug was prescribed.
- DO follow label instructions as to frequency, timing, and size of dose. Do not take a drug at random intervals, or on an empty stomach if "with meals" is specified (or vice versa). Do not "double up" if you miss a dose.
- DON'T drink alcoholic beverages while taking drugs unless your physician specifically says it is safe to do so.
- DO throw leftover or outdated medicines away promptly. Some become less potent, others dangerously more potent. Never save drugs for "next time."
- DON'T store similar looking pills in the same location or in same-color or same-size containers. Look-alike drugs are easily confused, especially at night or when you are tired, in pain, or under stress.
- DO be sure your doctor is fully informed of other medications you are taking—prescription or over-the-counter drugs—at the time he prescribes a new drug. Be careful not to mix medications without his knowledge and approval.
- DON'T store drugs where they may be damaged by excess

heat, cold, light, or dampness. Avoid cabinets in bathrooms that frequently get hot and steamy; do not refrigerate drugs unless specifically told to.

- DO call your doctor immediately when you experience an adverse drug reaction, develop unusual symptoms, or unexpected feelings.

HYPERBARIC OXYGEN. "Hyper" means increased and "baric" means pressure. Hyperbaric oxygen therapy (HBO) involves intermittent treatment of the entire body with 100 percent oxygen at above normal atmospheric pressures. While some of HBO's mechanisms as they apply to cardiovascular disease are yet to be discovered, it is known that HBO (1) greatly increases oxygen concentration in all body tissues, irrespective of blood flow; (2) stimulates the ingrowth of tiny new blood vessels to areas with reduced circulation, providing collateral circulation around an arterial blockage; (3) causes a rebound arterial dilation, an increase in blood vessel diameter greater than when therapy began, improving blood flow to compromised organs; (4) stimulates an adaptive increase in superoxide dismutase (SOD), the body's internally produced free radical scavenger; and (5) greatly aids the treatment of infection by enhancing white blood cell action, potentiating germ-killing antibiotics.

While not new, HBO has only lately begun to gain recognition for the treatment of chronic degenerative health problems related to atherosclerosis, senility, peripheral vascular disease, and other circulatory disorders. Where oxygen delivery to vital organs is reduced, common symptoms of occlusive artery disease, such as incipient gangrene, can be rapidly reversed with HBO.

Studies show that simply a couple of hours of breathing pure oxygen will speed artery cleanup. Chicago's Dr. Vesselinovitch demonstrated this beneficial effect of breathing oxygen with atherosclerotic rabbits who were given an "oxygen session" each day.

One of the world's most experienced authorities on hyperbaric medicine is Dr. Edgar End, clinical professor of environmental medicine at the Medical College of Wisconsin, who voiced his opinion on HBO's value for the treatment of stroke this way: "I've seen partially paralyzed people half carried into the (HBO) chamber, and they walk out after the first treatment. If we got to these people quickly, we could prevent a great deal of damage."

HBO is usually administered in a transparent, heavy-gauge

acrylic cylindrical chamber about 8 feet long and 3 feet in diameter. The patient, made comfortable on a cotlike stretcher, is rolled into the chamber, which is then sealed shut. While in the chamber, which is equipped with microphones and speakers, the patient can watch TV, listen to the radio, read, nap, or talk with the chamber operator or whoever is outside. During therapy, usually lasting one hour, the patient is surrounded by and inhales pure oxygen while pressure within the chamber is increased to twice the outside pressure, equivalent to what a diver would experience at approximately 30 feet below the surface of the water. At the end of the treatment, the patient is gradually decompressed to normal pressure.

It is only in the last few years that HBO has come to be used in conjunction with chelation therapy. Preliminary results are exciting. Patients with cerebral vascular disease recover from complications of strokes more readily when these two treatments are combined. Senile patients, including those with Alzheimer's type, respond better to both therapies than either one alone. The same holds true for gangrenous legs and feet caused by blocked circulation. HBO rapidly relieves pain, helps eliminate infection, and keeps the threatened tissues alive while chelation therapy gradually improves circulation. HBO is also an effective adjunct to other treatments, including surgery, drugs, and physical therapy.

The main drawback to HBO is the difficulty of securing treatment due to the extreme shortage of HBO chambers. There are estimated to be only 600 in the world and two-thirds are in Russia. Of those in the United States, many are huge, operating-room size, old-style chambers, which require an engineer and a crew of technicians to operate, making them so inefficient and expensive that most have been put out of service. When we were able to secure our HBO for the Mount Rogers Clinic in 1982, we indeed felt fortunate, since it was one of less than 40 installed in the free world that year.

SURGERIES OTHER THAN BYPASS. Great strides are being made in the development of competitive treatments to bypass surgery, many of them significantly less costly, simpler, and safer. Among the more promising advances:

PTCA (percutaneous transluminal coronary angioplasty): In this procedure (alternately called balloon angioplasty), a thin tube or catheter, with a tiny balloon at its tip, is snaked into a coronary (or other) artery, to the area of a well-defined blockage.

The catheter's progress is followed by direct visualization on a TV-like screen, so that it can be guided to the blockage. When the balloon is centered in the plaque formation, it is inflated, stretching the arteries. Since these blood vessels are not very elastic, they do not fully reconstrict, thus leaving a larger residual lumen (opening) than was there originally, freeing up blood flow.

While there is some theoretical risk of plaque breaking off or of the stretching process causing microscopic tears in blood vessel walls, neither has proved to offset the potential benefit.

Angioplasty, the hot new successor to bypass surgery, also has limited benefits. It may be highly effective for very localized lesions in accessible areas, as for blockages in arteries large enough to accommodate the catheter. Like surgery, the process can only unblock small segments of a diseased artery, and so may prove useless in patients where the disease has progressed too far, or where blockages are unreachable.

Laser surgery: Theoretically promising, this technique is in its infancy. But if all the technical problems can be solved, it has tremendous potential.

Once perfected, laser beams will be delivered via a tube containing super-fine glass fibers through the interior of clogged blood vessels, vaporizing obstructions caused by plaque directly, one by one. Researchers developing the process say they will be able to accurately and safely direct and adjust the intensity of the laser light to individual plaque requirements.

Still in the dry run stage, fiber optic experts, confident lasers will be the surgical tool of the late 1980s, expect to be vaporizing plaque clinically within two years. The problem of downstream embolization of plaque debris must also be solved. If so, laser surgery could eventually be a relatively minor procedure, administered on an outpatient basis. But it would still share the same drawbacks as angioplasty—useful only for accessible plaque.

Two other surgical procedures should be mentioned, although they do not counteract atherosclerotic disease:

Pacemakers: There is a world of difference between the first crude devices implanted two and a half decades ago and the pacemakers some half-million Americans depend on today to provide regular electrical impulses to hearts beating irregularly (too fast, too slow, or not at all). The newest versions of these life-saving devices, inserted beneath the skin of the patient's chest, with wires reaching to the heart, need little attention. They work on tiny, powerful, lithium batteries good for five or more years and can almost think for themselves. They are geared to adjust automatically to heartbeat malfunction and changing body demands.

For the small percentage of heart disease sufferers who require a pacemaker, it is a remarkable invention, but it has little to offer for the vast majority of atherosclerotics.

Heart replacement: Heart transplants were all but abandoned a decade ago, when most recipients survived only briefly. The operation, relatively simple to perform, was usually a success, but the patient died within weeks or months nonetheless, either because of organ rejection or massive infection. Between 1968 and 1983, new drugs, new tissue matching techniques, and new rejection monitoring techniques were developed, and when the one-year survival rate went from less than 20 percent to more than 80 percent, revived hope brought a new wave of interest. Some 250 operations were slated for 1983, with the number expected to more than double each year thereafter.

Researchers in the forefront of heart replacement technology now optimistically predict the procedure will be so routine within a decade or two that we will all line up for a new heart as soon as our old one shows signs of disease.

Adding credence to the prophecy was the Barney Clark extravaganza. When surgeons successfully replaced his ailing heart with what has been called the "Model T of artificial hearts" (implying useable replacement organs will be rolling off the production line someday soon), the significance of the accomplishment for the average heart patient was greatly overstated. Caught up in the euphoria of Buck Rogers medical achievement, it was easy to overlook reality and more dismal and sobering facts.

Donor organs are hard to come by. There are a limited number of young, healthy hearts, not injured by a death-causing accident. (An interesting sidelight: Early in heart transplant research, surgeons discovered they were unable to keep donor hearts alive and well unless they were immersed in a solution of EDTA.)

Transplant enthusiasts expect to lick the organ shortage problem by encouraging more public participation in donor programs, by perfecting xenografts (transplantation of organs from such animals as cattle and sheep), and by developing functional, practical versions of the artificial heart.

Say all that happens, will heart replacement then be a feasible alternative for masses of people?

Let's talk money. Should heart replacement technology be perfected, the costs—$50,000 to $100,000 per procedure plus $1800 to $8800 per year for ongoing care—would put it in the break-the-bank category, whether privately or publicly funded.

Let's pretend financial drawbacks can be overcome. Then can the average American hope to live longer by virtue of perfected new-hearts-for-old technology? Not even then.

Remaining is the drawback faced by most heart replacement recipients. They are stuck with the same old diseased arteries. The new hearts, real or artificial, may be capable of beating on indefinitely, but what use when patients have not been cured of their underlying disease?

The $200 million or more thus far devoted to the development of transplant technology has been badly misspent inasmuch as it is a piecemeal attack on the problem. Atherosclerosis affects the entire body, not just one organ, or one segment of artery. Heart replacements, like coronary bypass surgery, neither correct the precipitating ailment nor reverse its progress.

LIFESTYLE CHANGES. Improved diet, increased exercise, stress management, and giving up smoking and drinking, either alone or in combination with other therapies, have proven benefits. Most thoughtful researchers recognize that the advances in treatment for heart disease account for only a small part of the significant decline in heart-related deaths. Changes in health habits may be even more important. Record numbers of Americans have become "health nuts" in recent years. They're jogging, eating better, and buying nutritional supplements. As scientifically described elsewhere in the book, many vitamins, minerals, and trace elements are essential to the safe control of free radical reactions in the body. Vitamin C, E, beta carotene, and all anti-oxidants are free radical scavengers. Anything that will slow or control free radical damage is certain to slow the progress of degenerative disease.

Most cardiologists, whatever treatment they prescribe, prod their patients into adopting better health habits. My experience tells me that those patients who do adopt better habits undoubtedly do better, and thus they support the success rate of whatever therapy they're on.

All qualified chelation doctors consider lifestyle changes an integral part of the entire chelation program—so much so, that in my practice, acknowledgment is written into the patient informed consent literature.

In this category, there are lots of "right" things to do, and none of them will hurt you. While the evidence for benefit is not fully established, that is small reason to wait for all experts to agree on what may save your arteries—and your ilfe.

To emphasize how much importance we place on lifestyle changes for their potential to reverse as well as prevent disease, we are devoting two entire chapters to practical ways of modifying health habits.

One such approach, incorporating diet and exercise, deserves special recognition—the Pritikin Program, the brainchild of health entrepreneur Nathan Pritikin. A true pioneer, Mr. Pritikin, neither a doctor nor any type of health professional, but a genius and noncredentialed self-taught nutritionist, was the first to insist atherosclerosis could be reversed by following a stringent diet and exercise regimen. While most of the medical community laughed, he set about demonstrating he was right.

Hundreds of thousands of cardiac patients now believe in, and follow, the Pritikin Program. His claims of success are supported by numerous testimonials from men and women, many of whom canceled their scheduled bypass surgeries to give his diet and exercise regimen a try.

It is not easy to stick to the Pritikin Program. The diet, a very spartan high-complex-carbohydrate, low-fat diet that allows clients only 10 percent of daily calories as fat (the average American diet contains 40 percent of calories as fat), requires extraordinary discipline to abstain from your favorite "goodies," to give up smoking and drinking, and to exercise extensively.

Pritikin forbids eating all of the following: fats and oils, sugars, fatty meats, fried foods, shrimp, egg yolks, all but nonfat dairy products, jams and jellies, nuts, dried fruits or sweetened fruit juices, commercial products made of white flour or white rice, soda pop, coffee, tea, and alcohol.

As a reward, adherents to the program are offered the hope they will recover their health, and be pain- and symptom-free.

No matter how beneficial it has proven for some, the Pritikin Program is not for everyone. It is so extremely restrictive, with such rigid dietary restraints, that only a small percentage of people can sustain the cultlike devotion required for long-term compliance.

It is also extremely costly to get the full treatment at Pritikin's Longevity Center. Current charges are $4000 or more for only a month of lifestyle indoctrination, which does not include room and board for an accompanying spouse, travel costs, or loss of income during the prolonged absence from home.

Nevertheless, I believe all holistic-oriented physicians owe a debt of gratitude to Nathan Pritikin for popularizing a general approach we can all encourage in patients in a modified form. Of all the health gurus who have burst on the scene in modern times, I would credit Nathan Pritikin with having done the most good—and no harm.

And there is one final alternative:

NO TREATMENT. Rest and relaxation (R&R) may be all that is required for someone to go on living much the same as they did prior to their heart attack or angina pains. We have no statistics, of course, on people who opt for the hands-off approach to their disease, but suspect that some few may do as well as those who pursue the most aggressive avenues.

While I am clearly biased in favor of the therapies I know best, and have seen work so well for so many patients, I have no quarrel with people who choose to use other therapeutic means. I have no objection to surgery where clearly indicated and appropriate, but in my view, bypass surgery should be reserved until all nonsurgical therapies have been tried and found wanting. It should be the alternative of last resort.

14

Life After Chelation—Eight Things You Can Do to Live Healthier, Longer

How much longer do you want to live?

Ten, twenty, fifty years? Forever?

How healthy do you want to be?

Not such frivolous questions once you realize healthful life extension is within your control regardless of your current health status.

Not too long ago there was scant evidence you could forestall aging-related diseases, or reverse those already in progress. Now we know better. More than 80 percent of atherosclerotic disease is self-inflicted, preventable, and partially reversible. The "killer diseases"—cancer, included—are not the inevitable consequences of age, genetic background, or environmental exposure, as once thought.

You can live better, and longer, simply by altering lifestyle habits that subvert health and shorten life. The time has come to stop asking what your doctor can do for you (to paraphrase J. F. Kennedy) and ask instead what you should be doing for yourself.

Here are eight things you can do to maximize your longevity. Whether you adopt one, or all, the change for the better will move you closer to able-bodied condition.

1: Quit smoking.

Only a modern-day Rip Van Winkle, asleep for the past three decades, hasn't heard that smoking is a disease-producing, life-shortening habit. Even with all the warnings, the full hazards are not well known. It's not just the tar and nicotine content of cigarettes that will do in the smoker, but so long a list of poisons and toxic reactions, were they put on the package, there'd be little room left for the brand name. If you're still unconvinced, here is the newest damning evidence.

- Smoking greatly increases internal free radical production.

a) A pack-a-day smoker can absorb as much ionizing radiation in one year as he would were he to have 200 chest x-rays, according to University of Massachusetts doctors who have found radioactive isotopes, particularly polonium-210 (from phosphate fertilizers used in growing tobacco) and lead-210 "highly concentrated" on smoke particles. Radioactivity causes tissue damage by producing excess free radicals.

b) Tobacco smoke contains tars, free radical producing polynuclear aromatic hydrocarbons, that can cause genetic mutations that can result in cancer and the formation of atherosclerotic plaque. Free radical agents are absorbed from tobacco through the lining of the mouth, even when the smoker does not inhale.

c) Cigarette smoke contains acetaldehyde, a hazardous chemical cross-linker that causes undesirable chemical bonds between large molecules via free radical reactions. Abnormal cross-linking results in wrinkled skin and inelastic, hardened arteries.

d) Cigarette smoke contains heavy metals—lead, cadmium, polonium, and arsenic—that contribute to free radical pathology by limiting anti-oxidant enzyme activity and that poison metabolism in other ways.

e) Cigarette smoke contains carbon monoxide, which reduces the blood's oxygen carrying capabilities, and nitrous oxides, which increase free radical production.

- Tobacco triggers allergic reactions that can contribute to sudden death from heart attack.

A team of scientists at Cornell University Medical College found smokers and nonsmokers alike evidence allergic skin reactions to tobacco glycoprotein, an antigen found in tobacco leaves and cigarette smoke. Extreme anaphylactic reactions can disturb heart rhythms, weaken heart contractions, and interrupt coronary artery blood flow.

- Tobacco contains nicotine, which causes blood vessels to constrict, increasing blood pressure and reducing blood flow to vital organs.

"Pot" smokers are no better off, since they suffer the additional hazard of smoking paraquat-treated cannabis (marijuana). Paraquat toxicity speeds the cross-linking process.

My clinical experience adds another dimension. In almost every case where chelation therapy failed to improve a patient's health, he or she had continued smoking. In some instances, patients improved for a while, but their conditions worsened once treatments stopped.

Smokers can reverse damage by giving up their habit. In one California study of heart attack victims, most of those who ceased smoking had less evidence of arterial plaque within eighteen months to two years of the day they stopped. A Swedish study of men who survived a first heart attack comparing "quitters" with "nonquitters" revealed that those who quit had nearly half the death rate of those who continued to smoke. Other studies come to similar conclusions. The more time that elapses after your last smoke, the closer your coronary heart disease risk comes to that enjoyed by people who have never smoked.

2: Avoid smoke-filled environments.

"Pass-along" smoke is also deadly. Inhaling secondhand smoke makes the heart beat faster, increases blood pressure, and raises blood carbon monoxide levels. There is more cadmium, tar, and nicotine in the smoke drifting off a smoldering butt than inhaled by the puffer.

Those who insist on their right to smoke are infringing on your right to life. A recent Environmental Protection Agency study revealed the innocent nonsmoking bystander suffers damage equivalent to smoking four to twenty cigarettes a day. Children of smoking parents suffer twice the incidence of childhood ills—particularly respiratory ailments—as children of nonsmokers. If you live or work side by side with a smoker, as far as your lungs, heart, and circulatory system are concerned, you are a smoker, too. A study of nonsmoking Japanese wives revealed their health depended on whether they lived with smoking or nonsmoking husbands. Twice as much lung cancer turned up in women married to smokers.

What to do?

Encourage your employer, bridge club, and professional associations to adopt and enforce the "no smoking" rule, or segregate smokers.

When making hotel, restaurant, or airline reservations, specify the nonsmoking section.

If you cannot convince your mate to quit (or if you entertain smokers), equip your home with room air purifiers.

When in a captive situation, position yourself upwind of the smokers.

3: Get regular exercise.

The most exercise many Americans get each day is slamming the car door after parking as close as possible to the supermarket. Their motto: "Never take a step when you can 'let your fingers do the walking.'"

A growing subcult of exercise buffs ascribes to the opposite philosophy: "Don't walk when you can run." Some have developed jogger's addiction, the compulsion to run that five or more miles every day, come what may, including hurricanes, drought, pestilence, or alien invasion.

To what extent does exercise help the heart? There is conflicting evidence as to whether anything less than extremely vigorous physical workouts provide significant protection against heart attacks. Several studies suggest an athlete must "sweat" to substantially reduce the risk of myocardial infarction.

There is no argument that habitual, lifelong exercise is a plus. It improves the quality of life in many ways. It helps burn off fat, suppresses appetite, aids circulation, improves the HDL/LDL ("good" guy/"bad" guy) ratio in serum cholesterol levels, reduces anxiety and depression, and increases general fitness.

Anyone past their mid-thirties who has been only moderately active, however, would be wise to go slow before indulging in activities as strenuous as marathon running. At least one study has shown that half of sudden death heart attacks were immediately preceded by severe or moderate exercise. According to Dr. Meyer Friedman (of "Type A" fame), once someone has suffered a heart attack, he should refrain from strenuous exercise: he should not jog, run, play handball, racketball, or tennis.

What if you've always been a desk-bound exercise phobic who's hated the very thought of doing anything strenuous? Is it too late to start?

When a group of formerly sedentary men and women aged 60 and older were enrolled in an exercise program, it took only seven weeks for them to acquire fitness levels equal to average 40 to 50 year olds, according to Canadian researchers.

The best exercise? For anyone who feels up to it—or who works up to it—I recommend "wogging" (a term coined by Dr. Thomas W. Patrick, Jr., of Fort Lee, New Jersey). As the name suggests, "wogging" is the happy compromise between walking (not enough exertion) and jogging (too strenuous and joint-jarring).

To get the most benefit from wogging (which Dr. Patrick defines as "walking fast for pleasure, exercise and physical fitness, at different rates from brisk to rapid"), start off easy, about a block or two at first, and then work up to 20 minutes a day. This minimum amount of moderate exercise will help get more oxygen to more cells and that's a boost to the body's free radical defenses.

Almost as important as regular exercise is avoiding inactivity. Sitting down and relaxing while watching TV may be your favorite pastime, but two researchers have documented cases of blood clots brought about by long sessions of TV-induced immobility. Their suggestion? Get up and walk around the TV set every 20 minutes or so. The same good advice pertains to sedentary workers, whose heart attack rate has been found to be twice as high as employees in comparable, but more physically demanding, jobs.

When asked what he does to keep in shape, the director of the Cardiovascular Center at New York Hospital–Cornell Medical Center, Dr. John Laragh, reported that he believes in informal, nonstructured exercise that keeps the muscles loose, lively, and active. "You can do that around any office if you stay on your feet and move around," he said. "I rarely sit at a desk unless I'm writing. I use the stairs instead of the elevator whenever I can."

Exercise needn't be tedious. As Dr. Laragh said, you're not aiming at becoming a gladiator. Get fit for the fun of it, choosing relatively simple and pleasant ways to stay limbered up. You'll be more motivated to continue on a regular basis if your fitness regimen provides real pleasure as you keep your body in motion.

Among the things you might do to up your activity level: get a dog, go dancing, join a bowling team, health spa, aerobics class, or swim club, visit museums and art galleries, stand up and walk around while you talk on the phone, get rid of your remote TV tuner, do housework to music, park the car and walk, volunteer to tend a toddler once a week, team up with a hiking buddy, walk—don't ride—the golf course, disconnect telephone extensions at home.

4: Limit alcohol consumption.

To avoid health hazards, limit alcohol consumption to one ounce of pure ethanol per 24 hours (four eight-ounce glasses of beer, or three small glasses of wine, or two shot glasses of hard liquor). A relatively healthy adult can normally detoxify that amount of alcohol without exceeding the free radical control threshold.

Indeed, research conducted by the National Heart, Lung and Blood Institute suggests one ounce of alcohol a day may be good for your heart. Their long-term nationwide study involving thousands of adults confirmed a positive relation between limited alcohol consumption and favorable HDL levels.

Drink more than that, however, and you soon head for trouble. Alcohol is converted to acetaldehyde (closely associated with formaldehyde, or embalming fluid), which auto-oxidizes in the body in the presence of unsaturated lipids, damaging cell membranes in an explosion of destructive free radicals. Our bodies contain sufficient special enzymes to metabolize the acetaldehyde but this internal detoxification mechanism can be overwhelmed if too much alcohol is consumed at one time, or too fast, or if over the long term, heavy consumption results in free radical damage to the liver's enzyme production. Once acetaldehyde is left free to roam, it creates more and more dangerous free radicals, further hampering the body's built-in detoxification machinery, setting up a destructive chain reaction.

Avoid alcohol entirely if you are chronically ill or suffer serious degenerative disease.

5: Take a scientifically balanced nutritional supplement daily.

In the proper combination, supplemental nutrients will reinforce the body's natural anti-oxidant and free radical scavenging abilities especially when the supplements are taken with meals, that is at a time when the digestive process is apt to have triggered increased levels of free radical production. The product you select should protect against nutritional deficiencies and at the same time provide an adequate and balanced supply of those vitamins, trace elements and other nutrients necessary for protection against undesired free radical damage. To give you an idea of what to look for, six tablets a day of the product I recommend to patients, called Basic Preventive, to be taken two tablets at a time, three times a day directly after meals, provides the following:

Vitamin A	10,000 IU
Beta carotene	15,000 IU
Vitamin D	100 IU
Vitamin C	1,200 mg
Vitamin B1 (thiamine)	100 mg
Vitamin B2 (riboflavin)	50 mg
Vitamin B6 (pyridoxine)	100 mg
Vitamin B12	100 mcg
Niacin	50 mg
Niacinamide	150 mg
Pantothenic acid	500 mg
Folic acid	800 mcg
Biotin	300 mcg
Choline	100 mg
Inositol	100 mg
Para-amino benzoic acid (PABA)	50 mg
Vitamin E (d-alpha-Tocopheryl)	400 IU
Calcium	500 mg
Magnesium (aspartate)	500 mg
Potassium	99 mg
Iodine	244 mcg
Manganese (aspartate)	20 mg
Zinc	20 mg
Molybdenum (chelate)	100 mcg
Chromium	200 mcg
Selenium	200 mcg
Aspartic acid	816 mg
Bioflavonoids (Rutin, Hesperidin)	100 mg

This formula was devised with the help of a team of nutritional scientists, including biochemists knowledgeable about the complicated interrelationships among vitamins, minerals, and trace elements in metabolic functioning.

The tablets you take should be free of yeast, sugar, starch, artificial colors, sweeteners, or preservatives to avoid allergic reactions.

While proper nutritional supplementation is good, more is not necessarily better. Taken to excess, substances such as copper and iron, aside from being toxic, may speed free radical damage by catalyzing lipid peroxidation. The very elements essential for health and life are also potential health destroyers. Copper and iron supplements should be taken only with evidence of a proven deficiency.

The individual most apt to be at risk of oversupplementation is the true believer—the dedicated "vitamintologist" who avidly follows "panacea-of-the-month" revelations in magazine articles. Tinkering with nutritional supplementation is dangerous. Dietary micronutrients only work well in harmony with each other; a deficiency in one, or an excess of another, disrupts metabolism. For example, if you take high doses of zinc without copper, you may create a copper deficiency; take zinc without selenium, and you may increase the risk of cancer; take iron without zinc, you create a zinc deficiency.

Trace element supplementation, not a task for an amateur, should be under the supervision of a trained nutritionist, or knowledgeable health practitioner, who can tailor recommendations to individual needs based on dietary analysis, medical evaluation, and biochemical tests.

6: Learn to relax.

Do you plunge full speed ahead in a determined, forceful, never-enough-time manner?

Are you hard-driving, super-ambitious, goal-oriented?

Is your conversation full of "shoulds," "musts," and ought-tos"?

When there's a tough job to be done, are you the first to sign up for it?

While the connection between personality and coronary artery disease is not fully established, there does seem to be a certain type of individual (first described by Dr. Meyer Friedman and Dr. Ray Rosenman as "Type A's") that is exceptionally prone to heart attacks.

The typical Type A, according to researchers, is an intensely competitive overachiever, never satisfied with current accomplishments, always in hot and heavy pursuit of a more elusive goal. So-called Type A's, in the most extreme cases, are also aggressive, hostile, impatient, easily provoked, impulsive, argumentative, and bossy. As a class, those who fall within this category release more adrenaline and have a greater rise in blood pressure when stressed.

Type A's are not just high-salaried executives holding down

heavy responsibilities in high-pressure jobs. One study found 15 percent of stay-at-home housewives were Type A's and they, too, had twice the rate of coronary heart disease that Type B women had.

Animal researchers have discovered there are Type A bunnies. Fourteen rabbits were divided into two groups based on the way they reacted to minor stress. The "high stress" rabbits were found to have "significantly greater atherosclerotic plaque area than those rabbits which exhibited low stress," according to the report issued by the University of Southern California School of Medicine. They also had slightly higher blood pressure. In a yet more recent study, primates fed low-cholesterol, low-fat diets were divided into two groups—one group stressed, the other not. The healthy diet protected the unstressed animals from atherosclerosis, but not the stressed group.

If you're a Type A, chances are you know it. Friends, relatives, your children and your spouse are always urging you to relax and slow down.

Should you recognize yourself as being a Type A person, what can you do about it? Basic personality cannot be changed, but behavior can and should be modified. Behavioral change experts suggest trying the following techniques:

- Practice some form of relaxation.

It makes no difference what you call it—meditation, self-hypnosis, TM, mind control, or an altered state of consciousness. Each has proven benefits. If you have no particular liking for any structured relaxation technique, try 20 minutes a day in a hot tub letting your mind drift in pleasant daydreams. If you are religious, try prayer.

- Rid yourself of unnecessary and unproductive activities.

Delegate responsibilities. Learn to say "No" to requests you would prefer to turn down. Pretend you have only six months left to live, and set new work/play priorities.

- Free yourself from self-imposed time traps.

If you suffer from the "hurry sickness," with never enough time to get things done, chances are your problems are self-created. To break the time bind, stop wearing a watch; avoid committing yourself to closely timed appointments; do not schedule back-to-back activities. Develop the ***mañana*** philosophy. When things pile up, tell yourself, "Tomorrow is another day."

7: Expand and cherish your social network.

Science has begun to prove what was long suspected: The health of your heart depends to a large extent on the state of your emotions. While the body/mind connection has never been in question, only lately has it come to light that your best defense against a heart attack might come from maintaining strong, close, satisfying personal relationships.

One of the most startling—and convincing—illustrations can be found in the tale of Roseto, Pennsylvania, famous as the "town without heart attacks."

The story might never have come to light had not a local doctor, who had practiced there for 17 years, told several colleagues he had never seen heart disease in anyone under the age of 55. Temple University researchers found Roseto was indeed unique, virtually immune from heart disease, with a death rate from myocardial infarction less than half that of the neighboring towns, and half that of the rest of the country.

Scientists moved in to find out what was happening and thus began a 19-year study. For the first five summers, health professionals set up clinics and examined most of the over-25 Roseto population, recording histories, blood studies, urinalyses, blood pressures, and electrocardiograms. To their surprise, they discovered the Rosetoans—mostly Italian-Americans—were almost identical to people in neighboring communities. They were overweight, ate fatty diets, smoked, drank, rarely exercised, and had all the bad habits normally considered precursors to coronary artery disease.

Medical sociologists dug in, determined to find an answer. Finally, they came up with the one striking feature about life in Roseto which set it apart. In their published report, the scientists said:

"The people of Roseto adhered to a tenaciously held lifestyle, which reflected Old World values and customs. It was characterized by predictability and stability."

According to the researchers, Roseto was a town where everyone knew everyone else. It had a clannish quality. Family relationships were extremely close and mutally supportive. Neighbors helped neighbors; the elder generations were cherished and respected, and retained their authority throughout their lives; men and women held well-defined roles, and men were the uncontested heads of their families; personal problems were worked out within the family, or with the help of the local priest; social life revolved around the family, village celebrations, and religious festivals . . . until the early 1960s, when things began to change.

Some young people went away to college and never returned. The first generation Rosetoans began to die off. The birth rate declined. Church attendance went down. Interdenominational marriages increased. Rivalries cropped up. The more affluent began to show off their wealth. Men joined the country club; women slimmed down and dolled up. Fast-food drive-ins attracted the diners who formerly congregated at the five family-owned restaurants. The old, close, clannish feeling was gone, and beginning in 1966, there was a striking increase in death rates from heart attack. By 1975, Roseto's heart attack rate was identical to that of neighboring communities. What went wrong?

The doctors who followed Roseto's history believe it was the strong family ties, sense of community, and supportive social networks that once protected residents against coronary disease. As those bonds weakened, so did defenses against heart attack.

While we cannot recreate the Roseto that once was, we can recognize the value of love and friendship to our health and our lives. When Israeli doctors conducted a long-term study, they found a far lower incidence of heart attacks among happily married men who considered their wives loving, loyal, and supportive.

Loving and being loved is so crucial, it even extends to man's relationship with the animal kingdom. Psychologists studying the bond between people and their pets have discovered that men who had heart attacks, and owned a dog, were less likely to have a second heart attack than petless counterparts. Physiologists have documented beneficial physiological reactions when man and animal interact in a loving manner; pet your dog or cuddle your cat and your blood pressure goes down and your heart rate decelerates.

The implications are clear. Tender loving care must take its place along with the more traditional heart disease preventive measures.

8: Switch to a health-promoting diet.

We've left the best for last. The development of atherosclerosis takes decades. If the diet that produces this disease is changed to one that treats and prevents it, damage can be repaired and health restored. To help you achieve that goal, switch to Dr. Cranton's Anti-Free Radical Diet.

15

Dr. Cranton's Anti-Free Radical Diet

"The beginning of wisdom," says an ancient Chinese proverb, "is to call things by their right name."

Without question, the right name for this nutritional counterattack against atherosclerosis and cardiovascular disease is the Anti-Free Radical Diet. The name crystallizes the concept of combating the broad range of degenerative diseases by avoiding free radical producing foodstuffs and consuming an abundance of those rich in anti-oxidants and other essential nutrients.

Most people, of course, don't diet to get healthy unless they've been scared into doing so. They diet because they no longer fit into their best clothes, or want to be thin for a friend's wedding, or just cannot stand looking at themselves in the mirror anymore. Happily, the identical eating program that will prove a boon to your arteries and heart eliminates most fattening foods and so will also provide dramatic weight loss benefits.

This diet reverses free radical pathology, thus slowing the aging process, especially when it's in the earliest nonsymptomatic stages. It also helps you become slim and shapely as you are getting physically fit. You not only feel younger, you look it, too. Excess free radical activity causes the cross-linkages that "harden" arteries (it's the same process tanners use for curing animal hides into leather) and makes your skin look leathery and wrinkled.

If, as many leading researchers believe, it is excess exposure to both external and internal free radical bombardment from dietary and environmental sources and the body's own biochemical reactions that triggers the development of atherosclerosis (and accelerates all aspects of the aging process), then altering those lifestyle and nutritional factors that contribute to excess free radical production is the natural and sensible way to halt the pathology and undo the damage.

Recent discoveries in the field of free radical pathology have shed light on how free radicals work, where we get them, and how to guard against damage. As it turns out, some of the prime sources of pathologically active free radicals can be easily evaded via dietary manipulation. For example, we can avoid consuming processed unsaturated oils (particularly the more rancid ones) and stop eating highly processed foods stripped of essential protective anti-oxidants and other nutrients. We can also beef up our body's control mechanisms and anti-oxidant defenses by choosing foods that best neutralize free radical action.

This is a decided departure from the outmoded "no eggs, less animal fat" dietary approach to minimizing the risk of developing cardiovascular disease. Once a link between atherosclerosis and free radical pathology was established, the natural next step was to develop strategies providing nutritional protection.

Atherosclerosis, and related degenerative ailments, develop slowly over many decades. "Time is the great healer," wrote Disraeli more than a century ago. The Anti-Free Radical Diet provides healing time: it removes the dietary stimuli that promote free radical damage, giving the body a period of respite in which to repair and restore itself.

The Anti-Free Radical Diet establishes a five-pronged approach to combating free radicals.

- It reduces consumption of foods that metabolize readily into excess free radicals.
- It supplies optimal amounts of free radical scavenging nutrients.
- It provides ample quantities of those trace and ultra-trace nutrients necessary for normal metabolism—for healing, immunity, and the manufacture of anti-oxidant enzymes.
- It utilizes nonoxidizing food preparation methods to minimize free radical lipid peroxidation before consumption.
- It reduces intake of fatty foods with high caloric density, leading to reduction of excess body fat, and reducing internal sources of

lipid peroxide free radicals, while simultaneously improving appearance.

Unlike some rigidly restrictive nutritional regimens, the Anti-Free Radical Diet does not take all the fun out of eating. Nor must you swear off properly prepared eggs, butter, shrimp, liver, and other foods high in dietary cholesterol that have long been mistakenly maligned as potentially lethal.

It is not really a diet in the traditional sense, inasmuch as there are no meal plans to follow. It is instead an eating, cooking, and food selection program designed to help you eat "smarter." It can protect you against developing a free radical disease, or help you fight off further deterioration.

To live a longer, healthier life, build your nutritional defense around these guidelines:

• Reduce consumption of all dietary fats and oils, especially the processed polyunsaturated or hydrogenated varieties, to 20 percent or less of total calories consumed.

It's no news that today's typical American eats far too much fat, averaging more than 40 percent of total daily calories. That's easy to do. Fat hides in foods not ordinarily suspect. The diet-conscious individual who virtuously avoids gravy, fried foods, and mayonnaise may not realize that 40 percent of the calories in apple pie are fat, as are 63 percent of those in a sirloin steak, 78 percent of those in a hot dog, and 87 percent of those in peanut butter.

Although essential fatty acids are necessary for normal healthy skin, arteries, blood, glands, nerves, and all cells, most health experts agree on the wisdom of lowering total fat intake. They disagree, however, on how low is low enough. Some maintain no more than 10 percent—a truly Spartan requirement—of total calories is allowable; others say 30 to 35 percent is acceptable. My strong recommendation is to stay in the more easily managed 20 percent range, paying careful attention to sources, processing, and quality of fats and oils.

Moderating the amount of fat eaten is vital inasmuch as dietary fats are the prime source of excess internal free radical production. Fats fuel the body's metabolic free radical factory because of their chemical composition. Fats (especially polyunsaturated fats and oils) oxidize readily, triggering chains of free radical reactions.

The untold part of the fat story, however, is that reducing the quantity of fat is not nearly as crucial as eliminating the wrong kinds of fat. Contrary to current popular mythology, it is not the saturated (animal) fats that are the "bad guys" and the polyunsaturated fats (liquid oils of vegetables or seed origin) which are the "good guys." It is exactly the reverse if the oils have been exposed to light, heat, and air in the extraction, bottling, and food preparation process.

Saturated fats, as found in butter, eggs, beef, lamb, and pork, can be eaten more safely (when prepared properly), for truly saturated fatty acids are not peroxidized under normal conditions. In contrast, the polyunsaturated fats that are commercially processed (vegetable and seed oils) undergo extensive lipid perioxidation (with resulting damage to the molecular structure of the fatty acids), beginning the very moment these fats are extracted from the foods in which they naturally occur. Such chemically altered fats disrupt normal metabolism and when consumed, impair delicate cell membrane structures, initiating the mutation process that eventually leads to physical degeneration, plaque formation in the arteries, cancer, and arthritis. The richer the oil in polyunsaturated fatty acids, and the longer the oil was exposed to heat, light, atmospheric oxygen, and trace amounts of metallic elements, the more "rancid" (peroxidized) it becomes and the greater the health threat. The poorest quality oils are customarily used in the manufacture of salad dressings and mayonnaise, since their rancidity can be so easily masked by heavy seasoning. To compound the problem, the fat soluble anti-oxidant Vitamin E, which normally protects natural oils by retarding rancidity, is routinely removed during the manufacturing process to be sold separately as a food supplement.

Even the so-called cold-processed oils, premium priced at health food stores, are atherogenic. Just as soon as the oil is extracted from its source—the soybean, peanut, corn kernel, walnut, sesame seed, etc.—it begins to peroxidize.

Take peanuts, rich in both iron and copper, for example. When peanuts are crushed to make oil, or peanut butter, those trace metals are released from internal cellular compartments into the oil to become potent catalysts of lipid peroxidation. This increases the rancidity of the commercial product by a millionfold, all without the consumer being any the wiser. Unfortunately, extensive peroxidation can exist without a detectable rancid odor or taste.

Heating vegetables oils to fry foods greatly compounds the problem. When an oil is heated, the rate of peroxidation increases rapidly, doubling with every ten degrees centigrade rise in temperature. The chemical structure of the fat or oil changes to a form that further enhances the development of atherosclerosis. Hydrogenation, such as takes place during the commercial preparation of margarine, vegetable shortenings, and products like nondairy creamers and nondairy whipped toppings, also convert polyunsaturated fats and oils into dangerous products (trans isomerized fatty acids in addition to lipid peroxide free radical precursors).

Do you protect your family's health by substituting margarine for butter? Hardly.

Margarine is clearly more toxic. Contrary to what a popular TV commercial featuring an attractive Indian maiden would have you believe, by the time corn oil margarine reaches your table, it is completely unnatural. Not only have its original molecules been drastically altered, but its free fatty acids have been reacted with harsh chemicals. It has been treated by petroleum-based solvents and been "deodorized."

Here are some practical suggestions to help you keep your total fat consumption within safe levels:

1: When eating beef, lamb, pork, or veal, always select the freshest, leanest meat available. Aged meats owe their enhanced flavor to rancidity. Trim all visible fat before preparation. To satisfy your beef hunger, choose dishes such as casseroles or stews that provide smaller individual portions of meat than a roast or a steak. When a recipe calls for hamburger, precook it and drain off all the fat before adding it to the dish.

2: Frequently substitute fish and lean fowl for other meat. Even the leanest beef you can buy has more than twice as much total fat as skinless white meat from chicken or turkey. Remove as much of the skin and subcutaneous fat as possible before cooking or eating poultry.

3: Eliminate fried foods from your diet. Learn to become adept at greaseless cooking. Use nonstick cookware (Teflon is one popular, easily available brand), which never needs oils or fats to keep food from sticking to pots or pans. Slow-roast meats, fish, and fowl.

4: Use dairy products with the lowest fat content, such as 1 percent fat cottage cheese or skim nonfat milk. Cottage cheese and milk labeled as containing 1 percent fat by weight actually contain 10 percent of total calories as fat (a 2 percent fat product equals 20 percent of total calories as fat and so on).

Be wary of imitation dairy products. Pseudo-sour cream, for example, is often made with hydrogenated oils and has no place on this diet. Stick to fresh, natural foods as close as possible to the state in which they were grown.

5: Substitute vinegar, lemon juice, garlic, onion, or herbs for salad oils and dressings, tomato and other fruit juices for rich sauces and gravies. Garlic and onion have the additional benefit of being rich sources of dietary anti-oxidants.

6: Limit your intake of "hidden fats." Restrict your consumption of pies, cakes, puddings, ice cream, and similar desserts.

- Avoid like the plague the "white plague" foods—white flour, white rice, refined white sugar.

The American public now suffers from a form of "over-consumption malnutrition." Their diet contains too many calories that have been stripped by the food industry of most of the trace nutrients necessary for protection from external and internal pollution. The high-speed milling of grains such as wheat, rice, and corn results in the reduction or removal of more than 20 nutrients, including essential fatty acids and the majority of minerals and essential trace elements. Ideally, your refined carbohydrate intake should be zero—no breads, crackers, cereals, pastas, or snacks made from processed nutrient-depleted starches. Refined foods, including those misleadingly labeled "enriched," are seriously depleted of vital anti-oxidant nutrients.

For example, in comparison with the natural nutrients that exist in wheat grain, the percentage of each removed in the production of white bread, as best we can estimate, are as follows: 90 percent of the Vitamin A, 77 percent of the Vitamin B_1, 80 percent of the Vitamin B_2, 81 percent of Vitamin B_3, 72 percent of the Vitamin B_6, 77 percent of the Vitamin B_{12}, 50 percent of the pantothenic acid, 86 percent of the Vitamin E, 67 percent of the folic acid, 60 percent of the calcium, 40 percent of the chromium, 89 percent of the cobalt, 76 percent of the iron, 85 percent of the magnesium, 86 percent of the manganese, 71 percent of the phosphorous, 77 percent of the potassium, 16 percent of the selenium, 30 percent of the choline, and 78 percent of the zinc! At most, only four of these vitamins—B_1, B_2, B_3 and iron—are put back in the "enrichment" process. And iron supplementation has the potential to accelerate the radical pathology—if a deficiency does not exist.

Refined white sugar likewise lacks most vital nutrients, including the ingredients, such as chromium, needed for its own metabolism. Thus each spoonful you consume (the average American's annual sugar intake is more than 100 pounds) must "steal" the nutrients needed to break it down into a digestable form from other foods in the diet, or from reserves in the body's tissues. Insulin cannot mediate sugar metabolism in the absence of adequate chromium.

Many of the enzymes involved in free radical protection, such as catalase, superoxide dismutase, and glutathione peroxidase, require the very nutrients lost in the refining process. When functioning properly, these enzymes dampen free radical chemical reactions, allowing the desired biological effect without unwanted cellular or molecular damage. Without these control enzymes, free radicals can be generated at an ever increasing rate, damaging the body's cells, tissues, and organs.

In addition to enzymatic control of free radical reactions, there are many other molecules that neutralize unwanted free radicals on a one-to-one basis. These include beta carotene (pro-Vitamin A), Vitamin E, Vitamin C, the trace element selenium, and the amino acid cysteine. Without these substances (all virtually "zapped" out of natural foods during processing), the body cannot protect itself against undesired free radical damage.

The best way to cut down on your consumption of unrefined carbohydrates is to up your intake of natural, unrefined foods, particularly whole grain products and green and yellow vegetables, which should ideally make up about 60 to 65 percent of your total daily calories.

1: Read labels carefully. Choose whole grain cereals and whole grain breads; eat brown rice and whole wheat, buckwheat, or soy pasta products. Steer clear of products with the telltale "enriched" notation. So-called fortification does little to correct nutrient depletion. Labels can be very deceptive.

2: Cook from scratch. There are hidden sugars in hundreds of processed foods we don't normally think of as sweet—canned vegetables, salad dressings, catsup, biscuit mix, TV dinners, mayonnaise, steak sauce. Peroxidized and hydrogenated fats and oils are commonly found in factory-made and processed foods.

3: Avoid foods that contain these disguised refined sugars: sucrose, dextrose, corn sweeteners, corn syrup, maltose, invert sugar, raw sugar, brown sugar, turbinado, fructose. Most so-called raw and brown sugar is just refined white sugar, colored with a little molasses.

4: Be wary of sugar-free soft drinks or so-called diet drinks, especially those that are cola-flavored. They contain excessive phosphates, which disrupt normal calcium metabolism.

5: Eat mainly whole foods—fresh fruits and vegetables, whole grains, peas, and beans—whenever possible. Eat the food whole (the fruit, instead of the juice) and the entire vegetable (potatoes with skins). Train yourself to shop mainly around the fringes of your favorite supermarket, the outer aisles where fresh produce, dairy products, meat, and fish are sold. Avoid the inner sections, booby-trapped with brightly colored packages of highly processed foods.

- Increase dietary fiber.

Dietary fiber binds bile acids, which are the byproducts of the metabolic breakdown of cholesterol. By lending bulk to the contents of the intestines, dietary fiber promotes the speedier movement of bile acids through the digestive tract and faster excretion. This fiber-induced reduction of bowel transit time reduces the time that bile salts are subjected to putrefaction, oxidation, and reabsorption.

Sluggish bowels, often a direct result of eating too many low-fiber gooey, pasty, refined foods, allow bile salts to linger in the colon to become toxic and be reabsorbed, disrupting normal liver metabolism of cholesterol. As we previously described, oxidized cholesterol, bound to low-density lipoproteins, contributes to atherosclerosis and free radical disease.

Increasing your consumption of dietary fiber is easily accomplished.

1: Eat more root vegetables, such as potatoes (be sure to eat the well-washed skin), parsnips, cabbage (also high in natural anti-oxidants), yams, etc. Other high-fiber vegetables to make a mainstay of your diet are spinach, beets, Brussels sprouts, carrots, cauliflower, turnips, broccoli, and eggplant. (Carrots and yams are rich in beta carotene, a natural anti-oxidant.)

2: Eat whole grain bread, preferably four slices a day. There is very little fiber value to breads made of milled white flour.

3: Start every day with a high-fiber breakfast cereal (oatmeal, whole-grain or rolled wheat, millet, buckwheat, corn and barley grits). Be wary of the ready-to-eat varieties, which are generally low in fiber.

4: Add miller's bran to your favorite recipes. Whole bran granules have an innocuous texture and flavor that combine readily with the regular ingredients of a meat loaf, stew, or soup, without interfering with the taste or consistency of the finished dish. Be adventurous. Sprinkle bran on a salad, add it to your home-baked bread, stir it into a main dish casserole.

Good as it is, bran contains only one constituent of dietary fiber and is no substitute for a complete variety of whole-grain foods.

- Reduce salt consumption.

No matter how often you have been warned to cut back on salt, it is worth repeating one more time.

Cut back on salt!

Not simply because of the well-publicized link between excessive sodium intake and hypertension, or because salt increases body fluid retention, but also because cell walls damaged by free radicals lose some of their ability to maintain a proper sodium gradient. Excessive sodium leaks into a cell that is already compromised, causing further metabolic impairment. Small blood capillaries, damaged by free radicals, leak plasma into soft tissues, causing swelling and edema. A free radical-damaged sodium pump is less able to remove excess sodium from within cells.

Lowering your salt intake is easier said than done. Food processors add it to foods that rarely taste salty. For example, would you suspect salt to be an ingredient in Kellogg's corn flakes? Jello chocolate pudding? Low-fat cottage cheese? All three do contain salt, but the real surprise is how much. One serving of pudding contains 404 mg of sodium chloride (one-third the amount in a steeped-in-brine dill pickle).

Since salt is a likely ingredient in any processed food not specifically labeled "No salt added," here are the most practical ways to cut back:

1: Reduce voluntary salting. Do not use a salt shaker at the table.

When cooking, substitute garlic, onion powder, kelp powder, herbs, and natural spices in recipes that specify salt.

2: Limit your use of high-salt condiments—soy sauce, for example, and prepared steak sauces, gravies, and relishes.

3: Restrict your intake of salt-laden foods, including smoked fishes, delicatessen-style meats, canned soups, pickles, pretzels, potato chips, and similar snacks.

- Learn to cook the Anti-Free Radical Way.

More often than you might realize, it is not what you cook, but how you cook, that causes health problems. As a general rule, the faster food is cooked, the higher the heat levels at which it is prepared, and the more heat it is exposed to, the more health-destructive changes that occur. Heat speeds up the chemical reactions of peroxidation, which leads to free radical generation.

For anti-free radical cooking:

1: Limit broiling over hot coals.

If like millions of other suburban homeowners you relish backyard patio cooking, you will not welcome this news. Your cherished charcoal broiler is a potentially dangerous free radical generator. Charring food oxidizes it, producing free radical precursors, and this is the reason that charbroiled foods are carcinogenic. That sizzling steak (or hamburger, hot dog, chicken breast, or other meat), first well salted and seasoned, and then grilled to tasty perfection, becomes coated with dangerous compounds called "aromatic polynuclear hydrocarbons" (similar to those found in tobacco tars). These generate many free radicals, including singlet oxygen, the free radical against which the body has limited inherent defense. In fact, the smoke from a single steak's fat drippings contains as much benzopyrene as the smoke from approximately three cartons of (600) cigarettes.

Grilled hamburger presents a special problem. Because of its high fat content and the large surface area exposed to air and heat, it is the most easily oxidized of all meats. In addition, iron and copper (potent free radical catalysts) are crushed out of the meat's cells and into the fat during the grinding process, accelerating its oxidation, making it particularly dangerous, especially if the beef is a few days old.

The solution: Buy your hamburger fresh ground (extra lean) and use it at once. Or better yet, grind your own meat. Steer clear of fast-food burger servers.

Even if you can't give up your backyard grill—trim all visible fat from steaks, chops, ribs and both skin and fat from chicken.

2: Never, never fry foods.

The oxidation of the fat used in frying added to the oxidation of the fat found in the food itself add up to a double whammy. Even animal fats—chicken, pork chops, fish, or eggs—normally thought of as saturated, do contain unsaturated fatty acids and cholesterol, both of which oxidize easily.

Animal experiments have shown oxidized cholesterol to be so damaging that if as little as one percent of the cholesterol in your diet is consumed in its oxidized form, atherosclerosis may well be the result.

What does that mean in practical, everyday terms?

Eggs are okay, in moderation (just as long as your total daily fat intake does not exceed 20 percent of total calories), unless you fry them. Remember the 40 percent fat calories of eggs (2 mg of saturated fat, 200 mg of monosaturated fat, 200 mg of polyunsaturated fat, and 67 mg of cholesterol) contribute to overall fat intake. In its natural state, or when a fresh egg is either soft-boiled or poached with intact yolk unexposed to air, its cholesterol content remains unoxidized and is an excellent free radical scavenger. Quite the reverse is so when the egg is fried, scrambled, or cooked into a recipe. Then the cholesterol is oxidized into a number of cell-damaging, toxic byproducts. The same holds true for all animal protein foods containing preformed cholesterol, including most meats, many types of shellfish, poultry, and seafood. Fresh baked, poached, steamed, or microwave cooked with all visible fat removed, these are high quality foods; fried they become toxic.

Be doubly wary of restaurant fried foods, where highly oxidized (rancid) fat is often used over and over again. A diner risks being bombarded by free radicals that—as frequently happens—can result in a heart attack several hours after a meal laden with peroxidized, fatty fried foods is consumed.

3: Learn to cook without overcooking.

Easy advice to follow. Invest in a crock pot, a wok, and/or a microwave oven. All three methods rarely allow foods to exceed 212 degrees, the boiling point of water below which lipid peroxidation takes place more slowly. When using a wok, always add some water (not oil) to prevent food from getting too hot.

As for the microwave oven, contrary to what many alarmists have feared, it is your best protection against diet-related free radical damage, since it preserves anti-oxidants far better than many conventional cooking methods.

Studies of microwave cooking by independent university-affiliated home economists have confirmed the appliance's safety. Natural fats are not excessively oxidized; few polynuclear hydrocarbons or other dangerous residues are formed; the vitamin content of foods is well preserved.

4: Avoid using aluminum cookware.

Ordinarily, aluminum cookware would not be a problem because the human body normally does not absorb much aluminum. Recent studies indicate that aluminum does build up in tissues of some disease victims much more than others. Aluminum is widely used as a food additive. It's in our drinking water and in our medicines, and it's the dessicating agent that allows table salt to "pour when it rains."

Tissue rigidity from aluminum cross-linkages between large connective tissue molecules and enzymes damaged by free radicals is believed to be a complication of free radical disease. Aluminum deposition has been proven to occur in arteries of atherosclerosis patients and in the brains of Alzheimer senility victims and in some types of Parkinson's disease. Although this aluminum deposition in vital tissues may only occur after free radical damage is already present, it seems prudent to limit aluminum exposure whenever possible.

- Eat an abundance of fresh whole fruits and vegetables. Eat them as soon as possible after purchase.

While all methods of food storage result in critical nutrient loss, some are decidedly worse than others. Freezing food delays deterioration (provided the food was frozen immediately after harvest), but major nutrient losses can occur if the food is blanched prior to quick freezing. Frozen food continues to deteriorate with progressive lipid peroxidation even in the freezer, albeit more slowly. Prolonged storage, and thawing prior to use, also produces vitamin loss. The longer fruits and vegetables, whole grain products, fish, meat, and fowl stay on the supermarket shelf, or in your refrigerator or cupboard, the more nutrients lost, the less free radical protection they provide and the more free radical precursors that accumulate.

For instance, asparagus left unrefrigerated for three days prior to use (not unusual for a typical grocery store operation) have lost most of their B-complex vitamins before you ever get them home. The same holds true, in varying degrees, for store-bought lettuce, cucumbers, beans, peppers, onions, etc. This means, ideally, that you should buy only fresh-picked produce at farm stores and markets, and then buy only as much as you can serve and eat shortly after purchase.

Eat an abundance of foods rich in Vitamin C, beta carotene (pro-Vitamin A), Vitamin E, the B-complex vitamins, the trace elements selenium, manganese, potassium, and zinc, and other substances utilized by human cells to produce the dozen or more antioxidant control systems that regulate free radical reactions. Control mechanisms involve several enzymes, including catalase, superoxide dismutase, and glutathione peroxidase, and require Vitamins C, E, beta carotene, and trace elements such as selenium to be activated. Each molecule of mitochondrial SOD requires three atoms of manganese; each molecule of cytoplasmic SOD requires two atoms of zinc and one atom of copper; each molecule of glutathione peroxidase requires four atoms of selenium; catalase and peroxidase require trace amounts of iron.

It is because these nutrients must be present in sufficient quantity and in proper ratio to each other to activate free radical defenses that we place such emphasis on fresh, whole foods in their natural state. The most knowledgeable nutritional scientists cannot duplicate in vitamin/mineral supplements everything that nature provides in the proper order, proper ratio, bound to the proper substances, to do their proper job as free radical scavengers.

Also, iron and copper are potent contributors to free radical damage as catalysts of lipid peroxidation when consumed in excess of the amount necessary to activate anti-free radical enzymes. Copper and iron should not be routinely consumed in nutritional supplements unless biochemical testing indicates a deficiency exists, and then, only long enough to replenish normal body stores. A carefully selected diet containing a variety of unprocessed, unrefined foods will provide adequate iron and copper for most people. Special circumstances, such as excessive menstrual bleeding, chronic blood loss from the digestive tract, and malabsorption states may require long-term supplementation of iron (and possibly copper), but even then, periodic testing is wise to monitor replacement and avoid excessive accumulations.

You can get the highest concentration of Vitamin C from green peppers, broccoli, Brussels sprouts, cauliflower, strawberries, spinach, oranges, cabbage, grapefruit, and cauliflower. To beef up the beta carotene content of your diet, select lots of carrots, sweet potatoes, cantaloupe, apricots, peaches, cherries, tomatoes, and asparagus. The fruits and vegetables richest in the B-complex vitamins are peas, corn, potatoes, lima beans, and artichokes.

The rules to follow are simple to remember:

1: When shopping for food, give top priority to freshness. Of the alternatives, frozen should be second choice, provided you can be certain the produce has not been blanched or thawed and refrozen. Third place goes to dried foods. They deteriorate quite slowly, but lose most Vitamin C and Vitamin A content because of the high heat involved in the drying process. In last place, canned foods. Canning of fruits and vegetables causes the most nutrient loss—as much as 50 percent of such potent anti-oxidants as Vitamin C and B-complex vitamins—during cooking, alkali and acid treatments, and blanching.

2: Eat your vegetables raw when possible. Concoct your own nonfat salad dressings by combining whatever spices, herbs, and condiments you like with nonfat yogurt, nonfat buttermilk, and/or 1 percent low-fat cottage cheese. Most modern cookbooks have a variety of recipes for delicious oil-free salad dressings. When you must cook vegetables, undercook them. Steaming is less damaging than boiling.

3: Arrange to eat fresh foods within three days of purchase. Return frozen foods that reveal telltale refrozen signs when opened (food covered with ice crystals or a sheet of ice). Keep close track of food stored in your freezer. Check "use by" dates on containers (yes, they're often there, but you have to hunt for them).

4: Take a scientifically formulated nutritional supplement such as Basic Preventive . Whatever vitamins you choose, take them with meals. It is while you are digesting your food that vitamins are most effective because that is when their anti-free radical activity is most needed and that is when they are most readily metabolized.

Even if you eat a nourishing, well-balanced diet, rich in fresh, whole fruits and vegetables, whole grains, and lean protein foods, you will benefit from supplementation.

Depleted farmland will not yield sufficient nutrients, particularly trace elements, to keep your body's natural anti-oxidant defense system optimally effective. Much of what is grown on native soils is deficient in selenium, absolutely essential to the production of glutathione peroxidase, and chromium, without which carbohydrates cannot be properly utilized for energy by cells. Since neither chromium nor selenium are needed for the growth of plants, the agricultural industry has no incentive to replenish those elements in the soil.

Air pollution also contributes to selenium deficiencies. Sulfur compounds in the atmosphere that result from the burning of fossil fuels and that contribute to acid rains fall onto agricultural soils. Food plants will selectively pick up sulfur, if present in an abundance, rather than selenium, which competes with sulfur for plant uptake.

Not as coincidental as it sounds, many anti-oxidant nutrients vital to free radical protection also serve as weak natural chelators. Vitamins C and E, and the amino acid cysteine, help rid the body of toxic metals such as lead and abnormally located iron and copper, all free radical catalysts. Dietary supplements containing cysteine should be taken between meals, to prevent interference with normal trace element uptake, and not for long periods at a time.

- Avoid excessive use of Vitamin D-fortified foods—especially pasteurized whole milk.

Widespread food fortification with Vitamin D is now estimated to result in an average American intake of more than 500 percent the RDA (Recommended Daily Allowance). Vitamin D, added to animal feed, is passed on to humans in animal fat. Vitamin D in excess of the RDA contributes to abnormal soft tissue calcification, which is also associated with free radical pathology and aging. Virtually all dairy products are fortified with Vitamin D, even nonfat dried milk solids. Cholesterol oxidation products have Vitamin D activity that adds to an already excessive intake.

Whole milk contains 40 percent of calories as butter fat and cholesterol. Heating and stirring the milk during pasteurization speeds peroxidation of fatty acids and cholesterol, contributing to free radical disease. That is not true of breast milk or milk fresh from the cow.

- Avoid excess caffeine, soda pop, alcohol, and chlorinated drinking water containing chemicals.

Simply put, people fare better on caffeine-free diets. Drinking more than five cups of coffee a day considerably increases your risk of arterial disease and associated ailments. Caffeine results in an increased production of catecholamines (adrenalinlike hormones that produce free radicals when they are metabolized). With excess catecholamines comes free radical damage to nerve cells and nerve receptors, contributing to depression and other nervous system disorders.

Soft drinks, especially cola-flavored varieties (sugar-free or not) skew the body's delicate calcium/phosphorous balance, already a problem since the typical American diet contains twice as much phosphorous as calcium instead of the optimal one-to-one ratio.

Where does all the extra phosphorous come from? Red meats have many times more phosphorous than calcium, another good reason to rely on poultry and fish for high-quality protein. Almost all carbonated beverages have phosphate buffers to prevent the carbon dioxide from forming carbonic acid. Thirdly, extra phosphorous comes from processed foods laced with preservatives, many of which are phosphate-based.

Why is the calcium/phosphorous ratio so important? When it is out of balance, excessive calcium tends to leak into cells, deposit in soft tissues, and accelerate aging. When cells are overwhelmed by calcium, they die.

Two ounces of alcohol a day—no more—is a safe limit for most persons, except for pregnant women, people with seriously compromised health, and those with a predilection for alcoholism. Alcohol metabolizes to become acetaldehyde, a potent free radical precursor and cross-linker.

Water is no less important to our bodies than food, yet every day we have increased reason to fear the quality and safety of our water supply. In many cases, it is practically impossible to determine the composition of the water we drink. Public water supplies often contain numerous added chemicals that are possibly harmful (such as chlorinated hydrocarbons, which are free radical generating substances). Artificially softened water can also be dangerous because of its excess salt and occasional abundance of lead and cadmium, two of the more potent toxins and free radical catalysts.

The solution? Drink well water only when you are certain that the well is far away from any source of commercial toxic wastes. If you are suspicious of your local water supply, drink bottled spring or distilled water (not always reliably labeled, however). An alternative is to equip your tap with a tested and effective water purifier. Reverse osmosis water purifiers are quite good, especially in conjunction with activated charcoal.

When planning meals to suit the Anti-Free Radical Diet, here are the foods to include each day:

Vegetables. At least two *generous* servings of a variety of fresh vegetables, especially those known to be the chief food sources of the important anti-oxidants beta carotene (pro-Vitamin A), Vitamin C, and Vitamin B complex: artichokes, asparagus, beet greens, snap beans, lima beans, navy beans, broccoli, Brussels sprouts, cabbage, carrots, cauliflower, collards, chard, yellow corn, kale, kohlrabi, lentils, mushrooms, green peas, pumpkin, sauerkraut, snow pea pods, spinach, squash, succotash, winter squash, sweet potatoes, tomatoes, turnip greens, turnips, water chestnuts, and zucchini.

Salads. Two servings a day from any combination of raw vegetables. You can add extra anti-free radical potency by the liberal use of chicory, Chinese cabbage, cucumber, endives, escarole, lettuce, parsley, pimento, chives, red and green peppers, dandelion greens, watercress, radishes, scallions, garlic, onions, and leeks. Season salads with lemon juice, herbs, or oil-free dressings. Olive oil on salads is least likely to be peroxidized because it is a monounsaturate.

Fruits. Two to three fresh servings a day, not canned, cooked, or juiced, with the selection depending on individual taste and what is seasonally available. Chief fruit sources of anti-oxidant nutrients are apricots, bananas, cantaloupe, all melons, oranges, tangerines, papayas, peaches, plums, prunes, lemons, limes, pineapples, tomatoes, black currants, raspberries, rhubarb, and strawberries.

Protein foods. Two servings a day consisting of the following: four- to six-ounce portions of lean beef, pork, veal, or lamb, no more than two or three times a week. As often as possible, replace red meat with chicken or turkey, with skin removed. At least twice a week, choose a nonoily, white-fleshed fish (baked or broiled haddock, flounder, scrod, turbot, or water-packed canned tuna). Once a week, select an organ meat—liver, sweetbreads, kidneys, or brains.

Eggs. One or two a day, up to ten a week, provided you don't exceed total allowable fat, and as long as eggs are fresh-boiled or poached, with yolks intact, never scrambled or fried or cooked into other dishes.

Cereals and breadstuffs. Two to six servings a day (according to whether you want to gain weight, lose weight, or stay as you are) of unrefined whole grain products. These include such breakfast cereals as oatmeal, all bran, and shredded wheat, pasta, breads, muffins, or crackers made from whole grain flours, and brown rice. Breads may be sparingly spread with butter, never margarine.

Dairy products. One serving per day of one percent low-fat natural cheese, such as cottage cheese, farmer cheese, pot cheese, or skim-milk cheese. Drink only nonfat skim milk, two to three glasses a day.

Beverages. Decaffeinated coffee is fine (no more than three cups a day of nondecaffeinated coffee); herb teas—no restriction; milk—no more than three cups of nonfat skimmed milk per day; alcoholic beverages—limited to a maximum of 2 ounces of liquor, 8 ounces of wine, or two 12-ounce cans of beer; avoid all soft drinks. (The least harmful carbonated beverages are noncola, noncaffeinated, sugar-free diet pops.) There is no limit on naturally carbonated spring water.

Desserts and snacks. Choose fresh fruit, dried fruit, puddings, sherbets, and gelatins made at home from sugar-free recipes. For an occasional treat, have a handful of freshly cracked, unsalted nuts, fresh roasted chestnuts, dried raisins, or a slice of fat-free, home-made sponge or angelfood cake. Saccharine and aspartame in moderation as artificial sweeteners will probably be tolerated by most people without difficulty.

For rapid weight loss, restrict each day's food choices to the following for no more than two weeks without doctor supervision:

- Two small servings (4 ounces each) of lean white meat from fish or chicken, broiled, baked, or boiled with the skin removed. Flavor with lemon juice and add parsley. Use no salt, or very sparingly.

- No more than one egg a day, soft-boiled or poached.
- Drink only water, herb teas, black coffee (decaffeinated), or unsweetened tea (saccharine and aspartame are allowed).
- Start each meal with a salad, using unlimited amounts of any of the low-carbohydrate vegetables and salad makings listed below, seasoned with lemon juice, herbs, or nonoil dressings. The vegetables may be eaten in any quantity, cooked or raw as desired.

LOW CARBOHYDRATE VEGETABLES:

Asparagus	Chinese cabbage	Sauerkraut
Bamboo shoots	Eggplant	Snow pea pods
Bean sprouts	Kale	Spinach
Beet greens	Kohlrabi	String beans
Broccoli	Muchrooms	Summer squash
Brussels sprouts	Okra	Tomatoes
Cabbage	Onions	Turnips
Cauliflower	Peppers	Water chestnuts
Chard	Pumpkin	Wax beans
	Rhubarb	Zucchini squash

SALAD MATERIAL:

Celery	Endive	Onions
Chicory	Escarole	Parsley
Chinese cabbage	Fennel	Peppers
Chives	Garlic	Radishes
Cucumbers	Lettuce	Scallions
		Watercress

Take a high potency vitamin/mineral supplement such as Basic Preventive each day. Regular aerobic exercise will enhance well being and hasten weight loss.

Eating the anti-free radical way is not difficult, and very pleasurable. Learning to shop, cook, and eat so that your food intake enables you to be hardy and strong to a ripe old age is an exciting adventure. Adopting our nutritional guidelines is made more enjoyable by the knowledge that you have much to gain—a longer, healthier, happier life.

16

The Final Word— Take This to Your Doctor

Having read this far, chances are you know more about chelation than anyone in your neighborhood; sad to say, even more than your doctor.

No problem, until the day comes when you, or someone you care for, experiences the symptoms of cardiovascular distress (angina pains, breathing difficulties, a heart attack). Where do you go? To your doctor, naturally.

The truth is, you cannot chelate yourself. Nor can you turn to a chelation doctor to take over your total ongoing medical management. Your post-chelation health status may require the continuing surveillance of a primary care physician. Whatever treatment you choose, you will feel more comfortable with your doctor's approval and professional support.

No easy matter when chelation therapy is the issue. No matter how strong your present conviction that it has more to offer than other treatments, it is hard to stand your ground when your cardiologist's response to your question, "What about chelation?" is "Never heard of it," or "Thumbs down."

If you're like most patients, you'll feel trapped, cornered. You'll feel ill equipped to contest your physician's superior medical expertise, and fearful of antagonizing the specialist who may hold your very life in his hands. It takes a special kind of courage to tell your doctor you favor an alternative that he doesn't approve of and that has not yet become widely accepted by most physicians.

Some of my patients have resolved this dilemma by keeping their chelation treatments a secret. Others have changed doctors, more than once.

I believe there is a better way. Let us hope that your physician is a fair and open-minded professional, who understands the importance of keeping abreast of new developments in his field. Give him the opportunity to read for himself the latest scientific treatise (completely cross-referenced to over 230 articles from the world's scientific literature) on the causes and prevention of atherosclerosis and the rationale for treatment with EDTA chelation therapy.

Take this chapter to your doctor.

Free Radical Pathology in Age-Associated Diseases: Treatment with EDTA Chelation Therapy, Nutrition and Antioxidants

E. M. Cranton, M.D.
J. P. Frackelton, M.D.

An article in the Spring/Summer, 1984 issue of *Journal of Holistic Medicine.*

ABSTRACT: Recent discoveries in the field of free radical pathology provide a coherent, unifying scientific basis to explain many of the diverse benefits reported from treatment with EDTA chelation therapy. The free radical concept provides a scientific basis for treatment and prevention of the major causes of disability and death; including atherosclerosis, dementia, cancer, arthritis and numerous other diseases. EDTA chelation therapy, hyperbaric oxygen therapy, applied clinical nutrition, nutritional supplementation, physical exercise and moderation of health-destroying habits all have common therapeutic mechanisms which can reduce free radical causes of many age-associated diseases.

Elmer M. Cranton, M.D., a graduate of Harvard Medical School is a past Vice President of the American Academy of Medical Preventics; Past President of the American Holistic Medical Association; Charter Fellow, American Academy of Family Physicians; Diplomate, American Board of Family Practice; Diplomate, American Board of Chelation Therapy. James P. Frackelton, M.D., is Vice Chairman of the American Board of Chelation Therapy; Instructor in Chelation Therapy, American Academy of Medical Preventics; and past Chairman, Department of Family Practice, Fairview General Hospital, Cleveland, Ohio.

Elmer M. Cranton, M.D.
P.O. Box 44
Trout Dale, VA 24378
703-677-3631

Chelation therapy with intravenous ethylene diamine tetraacetic acid (EDTA) has been practiced by an increasing number of physicians for over three decades. Published studies describe beneficial results using intravenous EDTA as therapy for patients with chronic degenerative diseases.[1-47] Reports of renal injury and other adverse effects from this therapy are now known to have been caused by doses exceeding 50 mg/Kg/day, by pre-existing kidney disease and by heavy metal toxicity.[48-56] No published studies utilizing currently accepted treatment procedures contain negative data. The oft cited Kitchell report contained a negative conclusion,[57] although the hard data was quite favorable to the therapy. A careful review[58] of the data in that report does not support the negative conclusion. Research with laboratory animals provides further support for the effectiveness of EDTA chelation therapy.[59-65]

FREE RADICAL CAUSES OF DEGENERATIVE DISEASE

Recent discoveries in the field of free radical pathology provide a coherent and scientific basis to explain many of the reported benefits resulting from EDTA chelation therapy, usually in conjunction with nutritional and life-style changes. The field of free radical biochemistry is as revolutionary and profound in its implications for medicine as was the germ theory and science of microbiology which made possible development of effective treatments for infectious diseases. The free radical concept explains contradictory epidemiologic and clinical observations and provides a scientific basis for treatment and prevention of many of the major causes of long-term disability and death—atherosclerosis, dementia, cancer, arthritis and other age-related diseases.[66-75]

Methods for the detection and measurement of free radicals have only recently been developed.[76-78] EDTA chelation therapy and hyperbaric oxygen therapy, when properly administered in a program of physical exercise, applied clinical nutrition and moderation of health-destroying habits, all have common therapeutic mechanisms which reduce free radical damage.

WHAT ARE FREE RADICALS?

Free radicals are promiscuously reactive molecules and molecular fragments which react aggressively with other molecules rapidly creating new carbon-carbon and carbon-hetero-atom bonds.[79] A free radical has an unpaired electron in an outer orbit, causing it to be highly unstable and to react almost instantaneously with any substance in its vicinity.[80] The half life of a biologically active free radical is measured in microseconds.[68] This reaction often produces a cascade of free radicals in a multiplying effect.[66, 69, 70, 77, 79, 81, 82] Harmful effects of high-energy ionizing radiation (ultraviolet light, x-rays, gamma rays, cosmic radiation) result because photons of radiation knock electrons out of orbiting pairs, creating free radicals in living tissues.[78, 83-87] Free radicals in cell membranes produce pathologic oxyarachidonic and oxycholesterol products.[66, 87-90] Protection against pathologic free radicals is provided by dietary and endogenous antioxidants.[66, 67, 71, 73, 74, 91, 92]

Many free radical chemical reactions occur normally in the body and are necessary for health.[66-68, 71, 73-75, 93-96] This process might be thought of as a form of controlled "internal radiation." Highly reactive free radical molecules which are continuously produced within human cells include hydroxyl radicals, superoxide radicals, and excited or singlet state oxygen.[67-75] Free radicals react to produce hydrogen peroxide and other peroxides which are metastable, highly reactive molecules that rapidly produce additional organic free radicals in biologic tissues.[79, 80] To prevent uncontrolled multiplication of free radicals, human cells utilize more than a dozen antioxidant control systems which regulate the desirable free radical reactions.[66-69, 71-74, 77, 78, 84, 89, 91, 97-102]

Control mechanisms involve several enzymes, including catalase, superoxide dismutase and glutathione peroxidase, in conjunction with vitamins C, E, beta carotene, the trace element selenium and others. When functioning properly, these antioxidant systems suppress excessive free radical reactions, allowing healthful biological effects without unwanted cellular and molecular damage. Without these control systems free radicals multiply rapidly, much like a nuclear chain reaction, disrupting cell membranes, damaging enzymatic proteins, interfering with both active and passive transport across cell membranes and causing mutagenic damage to nuclear material. An abnormally functioning or malignant cell may result.[66, 69, 70, 77, 81, 82, 103, 104]

The concentration of the free radical control enzyme superoxide dismutase (SOD) in various mammalian species is directly proportional to their life spans. Humans have the highest concentration of

SOD. It is the fifth most prevalent protein molecule in the human body.[69, 70] Life expectancy therefore seems highly dependent on effective free radical regulation.

There are a number of non-enzymatic free radical scavengers, some of which can be stoichiometrically consumed on a one-to-one ratio when neutralizing free radicals. These include beta carotene (pro-vitamin A); vitamin E; vitamin C; glutathione; cysteine, methionine, tyrosine; cholesterol; glucocorticosteroids and selenium.

Enzymes involved in free radical protection require trace elements or B vitamins as co-enzymes. The trace elements copper, zinc and manganese are essential to the superoxide dismutases; selenium is essential to glutathione peroxidase; and iron is necessary for catalase and some forms of peroxidase. Adequate dietary intake of these trace elements is necessary for protection against free radical produced disease.

IDENTIFYING FREE RADICALS

Free radicals are highly unstable. They react rapidly in living tissues and therefore have a low steady state concentration. They rarely reach levels sufficient for direct analysis.[66] Newly developed instruments have revealed the importance and extent of free radical damage in tissues. It is now possible to detect the presence of free radicals using electron paramagnetic resonance spectroscopy (EPR).[77, 78] However, their effects can be measured more precisely by analysing the end products of free radical reactions, using gas chromatography, mass spectroscopy and high-performance liquid chromatography. Cross-linkages, damaged collagen, lipid peroxides, oxyarachidonate, oxidized cholesterol, mucopolysaccharide breakdown products, lipofuscin, ceroid and increased melanin all result from undesirable free radical reactions and can be readily quantitated.[66, 69, 70, 78, 105, 106]

By sifting through molecular wreckage left in the wake of free radicals, it is possible to determine the type and extent of ongoing free radical reactions. For example, free radicals in the central nervous system (CNS) can be assessed by the rate of disappearance of cholesterol. Cholesterol has no degradation enzyme in the central nervous system. The only way for cholesterol to diminish in the CNS is through auto-oxidation caused by free radicals.[69, 70, 107, 108]

CHOLESTEROL METABOLISM

Cholesterol is an antioxidant and free radical scavenger which protects cell membranes. It is liberally disbursed in cell walls, protecting vital phospholipids from free radical damage.[78, 107, 109] Cholesterol also acts as a precursor to the many steroid hormones and vitamin D. Vitamin D is normally produced in the skin by exposure of cholesterol to ultraviolet radiation from sunlight. Ultraviolet light is a form of ionizing radiation which produces free radicals in living tissues.

Total cholesterol (reflected by blood cholesterol) is determined primarily by cholesterol synthesis in response to ongoing oxidative stress from free radicals, not primarily by dietary cholesterol intake. Serum cholesterol levels are indicators of free radical damage and therefore correlate with the risk of atherosclerosis.[66, 69, 70, 78, 110] Cholesterol is synthesized in the body as needed and the need is greater in those at risk. In Western cultures affected with epidemic free radical diseases, blood cholesterol levels increase with age. Subsequent alterations of LDL receptor sites and underlying hereditary factors also cause blood cholesterol to rise.

Free radicals oxidize and peroxidize cholesterol into a variety of degradation products.[66, 68, 69, 78, 109, 110] Oxidized cholesterol is bound selectively to low density lipoproteins as LDL cholesterol while unoxidized (antioxidant) cholesterol is bound to high density lipoproteins as HDL cholesterol.[69, 70] The oxidation of cholesterol results in end-products with varying toxicity.[66, 110–112] Some of these products have vitamin D activity which causes localized vitamin D excess in tissues and macrophages.[110] Calcium is deposited in response to the resulting excess of vitamin D. Free radicals also increase tissue calcium by damaging the integrity of cell membranes and by impairing active transport mechanisms.

Dietary restriction of cholesterol and medications to reduce blood cholesterol have been counterproductive in the treatment of atherosclerosis because the antioxidant role of cholesterol has not been recognized. Unoxidized cholesterol is widely dispersed in cell membranes as a protective factor against atherosclerosis, cancer and other free radical induced diseases. In its antioxidant form it is not the harmful substance we have been led to believe. Cholesterol is fat soluble and restriction of dietary cholesterol therefore results in a reduction of total dietary fats. This is beneficial not because of cholesterol restriction (unless the cholesterol has been oxidized prior to consumption in food processing as is often the case), but because of reduced intake of lipid peroxide-containing fats and resulting in reduction of free radical pathology.

Statistics correlate very low blood cholesterol levels with an increased risk of some types of cancer. If adequate amounts of cholesterol cannot be produced, because of nutritional or metabolic factors, an effective defense against free radical causes of cancer has been lost. Free radicals are both primary initiators and subsequent promoters of malignant change. High fat diets rich in lipid peroxides are a major cause of cancer.[66, 69, 70]

A number of other cholesterol-derived steroids such as glucocorticosteroids, dehydroepiandrosterone (DHEA) and estrogen are also effective free radical scavengers.[78] DHEA and estrogen both diminish rapidly in middle age, a time when free radical related diseases accelerate.

ESSENTIAL FREE RADICAL REACTIONS

Human life cannot exist without a balance of carefully regulated free radical reactions. Organisms which live in the presence of oxygen must have free radical protection or they quickly die. Cellular respiration requires transfer of electrons across mitochondrial membranes. A superoxide radical is produced for each electron transferred. These superoxide radicals are quickly neutralized by mitochondrial superoxide dismutase (SOD), a manganese-containing enzyme. (The average American diet contains sub-optimal amounts of manganese.[113]) SOD elsewhere in cellular cytoplasm contains zinc and copper (also marginal to deficient in many American diets).[113]

Detoxification of many chemicals including drugs, artificial colorings and flavorings, petrochemicals and chemical fumes is performed in the endoplasmic reticulum of liver cells and other organs by cytochrome P-450 enzymes. This detoxification reaction produces both hydroxyl-free radicals and peroxides.[66, 93-95] Adequate glutathione peroxidase and vitamin C must be present to prevent free radical proliferation. Increasing exposure to drugs and chemicals causes increased production of free radicals to a point which exceeds the threshold of antioxidant protection. Excess free radicals then proliferate in chain reactions, multiplying their damage by a million times or more.[66, 70]

Synthesis of prostaglandins and leukotrienes from unsaturated fatty acids also results in release of free radicals.[70, 74, 96] Conversely, in the presence of excessive free radicals, the synthesis of prostaglandins may be imbalanced. For example, production of thromboxane increases while prostacyclin decreases in the presence of lipid peroxides.[66, 69, 70, 114]

Leukocytes and macrophages are potent generators of free radicals. Disease-causing organisms are destroyed by free radicals which are used much like "bullets" by macrophages.[115, 116] This might be compared to the concept of "limited nuclear war." Free radical production must be contained within the leukocytes. If the threshold of control is exceeded, free radicals proliferate into adjacent tissues, resulting in explosive chain reactions producing a million or more free radicals for each free radical which escapes. Clinically this is seen as inflammation.

Without antioxidant enzymes we would die instantly. With reduced amounts the aging process accelerates.[66, 69, 70] A graphic clinical example of accelerated aging is the disease known as progeria caused by hereditary absence of free radical protective enzymes. Within 10 to 15 years of birth, a victim of this disease proceeds through every aspect of the aging process including wrinkled, dried and sagging skin; baldness; bent and frail body; arthritis; and advanced cardiovascular disease. One form of progeria has been successfully treated by administering the free radical protective enzyme catalase. Hereditary traits vary widely throughout the population, even in those without progeria, determining each individual's unique resistance to free radical diseases. Some people can tolerate much more dietary and life-style abuse than others.

OXYGEN TOXICITY

Ongoing free radical pathology is often referred to as "oxidative stress." Ground state or unexcited atmospheric oxygen has the unique property of being a free radical generator and a free radical scavenger.[66, 117, 118] A liter of normal atmospheric air on a sunny day contains over one billion hydroxyl free radicals.[90] Oxygen at normal physiologic concentrations neutralizes more free radicals than it produces.[119] When oxygen tension is reduced, as occurs in an ischemic organ, oxygen becomes a net contributor to free radical damage.[69, 70, 120] Yet, without oxygen, life could not proceed at all.

Oxygen in high concentrations for prolonged periods of time can cause severe toxicity and death, primarily by free radical damage to the lungs and brain. Under proper conditions intermittent high pressure oxygen administered for short periods in a hyperbaric (HBO) chamber can stimulate repair of free radical damage and cause an adaptive increase of superoxide dismutase.[118, 121]

FREE RADICAL PROTECTION

Proper oxygenation enhances free radical defenses. Aerobic exercise stimulates blood flow and improves oxygen utilization, resulting in adequate oxygenation to remote capillary beds. When proper conditions exist, oxygen acts as a free radical scavenger and reduces free radical pathology.

We have already described the essential and desirable role played by nutritional trace elements which activate antioxidant enzyme systems. Each molecule of mitochondrial SOD contains three atoms of manganese. Each molecule of cytoplasmic SOD contains two atoms of zinc and one atom of copper. Each molecule of glutathione peroxidase contains four atoms of selenium. Catalase and peroxidase contain iron. Elemental selenium is also an antioxidant, independent of its function as a co-enzyme.

The human body lacks an effective enzymatic defense against the very destructive free radical precursor, excited state singlet oxygen. When superoxide radicals exceed the control threshold of superoxide dismutase (SOD), they spontaneously produce singlet oxygen. Polynuclear aromatic hydrocarbons (PAH) and aldehydes found in tobacco tar and tobacco combustion products produce a variety of free radicals, often mediated by singlet oxygen. The most important protection against singlet oxygen is dietary intake of beta carotene (pro-vitamin A), the yellow pigment found in carrots and other fruits and vegetables.[122, 123] Recent epidemiologic evidence correlates increased dietary beta-carotene with reduced incidence of cancer, even in smokers. Fully active vitamin A lacks this protective activity.[66, 69, 70] Vitamin E (tocopherol), vitamin C (ascorbate), selenium in glutathione peroxidase, the amino acid cysteine in reduced glutathione, vitamin B_2 (riboflavin), and vitamin B_3 (niacin) are all interrelated in a stepwise, sequential recycling process which provides ongoing neutralization of free radicals. If each one of these nutrients is present in adequate amounts, they can all be restored to their active antioxidant forms after reacting with free radicals. The process proceeds as follows: vitamin E neutralizes a free radical by oxidizing to tocopherol quinone. Tocopherol quinone is recycled to reduced vitamin E (tocopherol) by vitamin C, which is in turn oxidized to dehydroascorbate. Interestingly, the ratio of ascorbate to dehydroascorbate diminishes progressively with age and no specie of animal survives when that ratio falls below one to one.[70] Oxidized (dehydro) vitamin C is then recycled to ascorbate by glutathione peroxidase. Glutathione peroxidase is returned to its active form by oxidation of reduced glutathione. Oxidized glutathione is then reduced by the vitamin B_2-dependent enzyme, glutathione reductase. Glutathione reductase is reactivated by vitamin B_3-containing reduced NADH. Oxidized NAD is handed off to the Krebs cycle where residual energy, which originated with a free radical, is utilized for desirable metabolic purposes. These subsequent steps in energy metabolism utilizes a variety of trace element and vitamin dependent enzymes. From this stairstep cycle of oxidation-reduction reactions it is obvious that continued activity of each antioxidant depends on an adequate supply of the next antioxidant in sequence.[92] This interdependence explains the often equivocal results obtained from clinical trials utilizing only one antioxidant alone.

If free radical production exceeds the control threshold of this sytem, other antioxidant mechanisms must compensate. If other mechanisms are not adequate, serious damage to cell membranes, protein molecules and nuclear material results.[66, 79, 87, 89, 91]

An understanding of free radical defenses provides a scientific basis for nutritional supplementation with vitamins and trace elements, in safe amounts and in proper physiologic ratios—including vitamin E, beta carotene, vitamin C, glutathione, and B-complex vitamins. Although high levels of most water-soluble vitamins are rapidly excreted, transient tissue elevations do enhance free radical protection and other metabolic functions.

INCREASED PRODUCTION OF FREE RADICALS

When free radicals in living tissues exceed safe levels, the result is cell destruction, malignant mutation, tumor growth, damage to enzymes and inflammation, which manifest as age-related, chronic degenerative diseases. Each uncontrolled free radical multiplies by a million-fold.[66-70, 79, 87, 89, 91]

Dietary fats, especially polyunsaturated fats, are the leading sources of pathological free radicals. Unsaturated double-bonds on polyunsaturated fatty acids combine spontaneously with atmospheric oxygen, creating lipid peroxides. Polyunsaturated fatty acids are the "kindling wood" of smoldering free radical reactions in cellular membranes.[66]

Lipid peroxidation occurs as soon as fats and oils are extracted from the foods in which they naturally occur. Oxidative damage to dietary fats and oils is catalyzed by metallic ions, especially iron and copper. For example, peanuts crushed to make peanut butter are rich in both iron and copper which are released into the polyunsaturated oil when the peanut is disrupted. Iron and copper are potent catalysts of lipid peroxidation and increase the rate of rancidity of peanut oil by a million times. Massively peroxidized lipids are called "rancid." However, very extensive peroxidation can exist without a detectable rancid odor or taste.[69, 70] Extensive lipid peroxidation inevitably results during the manufacture of peanut butter. The same is true of most other salad and cooking oils, even so-called cold-pressed oils.

The richer the oil in polyunsaturated fatty acids, the more rapidly peroxidation will occur. The rate of peroxidation is proportional to the square of the number of unsaturated bonds on each fatty acid molecule. Other factors which increase the rate of peroxidation of dietary fats and oils include heat, atmospheric oxygen, light and trace amounts of unbound metallic elements.[69, 70, 87] Oils prepared in the dark, without heat, in an atmosphere of pure nitrogen, containing fat-soluble antioxidants such as vitamin E, would be the safest for nutritional use. Such oils are not commonly feasible.

Polyunsaturated vegetable oils containing iron and copper catalysts are routinely exposed to heat and oxygen when frying foods. This is the worst possible combination. Salad oils and oils used in the manufacture of salad dressings such as mayonnaise contain very high concentrations of lipid peroxides. The poorest quality oils are customarily used because rancidity is masked by heavy seasoning.

Peroxidation and hydrogenation of vegetable oils during the

manufacture of margarine and shortening also results in cis to trans isomerization. Transisomerization alters the three-dimensional configuration of dietary fatty acids from their normal cisoid coils to straightened transoid chains. Trans-fatty acids are incorporated into cell membranes in the place of naturally occurring cis forms, causing impairment of membranes and altering the function of phospholipid-dependent enzymes contained in cell membranes.[66, 69, 124, 125] Substrate recognition by enzymes which synthesize cell membranes is not adequately discriminating to distinguish between these two stereo isomers.[70] Phospholipids in cell membranes are damaged by free radicals. The process is initiated by dietary intake of peroxidized fats. Arachidonic and linoleic acids, both prostaglandin precursors, are lost in the process. These losses can be measured by gas chromatography. Cell membranes containing transoid fatty acids have altered fluidity characteristics which increase their permeability and interfere with active transport enzymes for sodium, potassium, calcium, magnesium and other substances. Adverse effects from transisomerization of fatty acids is additive to the other adverse effects of lipid peroxidation.[66, 69, 70]

Very little attention has thus far been given to the quality of dietary fats and oils. The emphasis has mistakenly been placed on the ratio of saturated to polyunsaturated fatty acids, irrespective of lipid peroxidation and cis- to trans- isomerization. We now know that the polyunsaturated fats are relatively more toxic. Margarine contains far more peroxides and transisomerized fatty acids than butter although limiting dietary consumption of all fats and oils is desirable.[70]

Excessive dietary fat is the most important cause of free radical pathology—not the ratio of polyunsaturates to saturates.[66, 69, 70] If dietary fats and oils are obtained from fresh, whole, unfractionated, unprocessed foods, they will not be peroxidized and will form healthy cell membranes with normal cis-configurations and result in a normal balance of prostaglandins. Although fully saturated fats are not subject to lipid peroxidation, all animal fats contain some polyunsaturated fatty acids and cholesterol, both of which undergo auto-oxidation. Animal experiments have shown that if as little as 1% of dietary cholesterol is consumed in its oxidized form, atherosclerosis may result.[110, 111, 126]

How much fat can the human body tolerate? Evidence indicates that the average person can safely consume 20 percent of dietary calories as commercially available fat without exceeding the control threshold of endogenous free radical protection.[69, 70] The quality of dietary fats and oils can increase or decrease this percentage. The average American now consumes in excess of 40% of calories as fat, mostly of poor quality with no consideration for rancidity. Lipid peroxidation occurs even when foods are frozen, although more slowly.[70]

Lecithin is a phospholipid rich in polyunsaturated fatty acids. Analysis of all commercially available lecithin indicates a high degree of peroxidation. The only way to extract lecithin without extensive peroxidation is in an atmosphere of 100 percent nitrogen, a prohibitively costly process.[70]

Research into senility, dementia, brain ischemia, stroke and spinal cord injury provides a wealth of evidence to incriminate free radicals as a cause of nervous system disease and provides a rationale for future treatment. The brain and spinal cord contain the highest concentration of fat of any organ. Central nervous system fats are also rich in highly unsaturated arachidonic and docosahexanoic acids. As previously stated, lipid peroxidation increases exponentially with the number of unsaturated double bonds per fatty acid molecule. Docosahexanoic and arachidonic acids will peroxidize many times more readily than other lipids. It is therefore necessary for the central nervous system to have additional protection against free radicals. Vitamin C is highly concentrated in the brain by a metabolically active pump. Ascorbate is 100 times more concentrated in the central nervous system than in most other organs.[70] There are two ascorbate pumps in series. The first increases the concentration ten-fold from blood to cerebrospinal fluid. A second pump extracts cerebrospinal fluid ascorbate and concentrates it by another factor of ten surrounding neurones of the brain and spinal cord. The primary function of this vitamin C is to protect fats in nerve tissue from peroxidative damage. The disappearance rate of vitamin C from the central nervous system is used as an indicator of the rate of lipid peroxidation following ischemia or trauma.[127, 128]

Observations of experimental spinal cord injury provide further support for treatments aimed at free radial protection. In animal experiments it has been shown that even a minor contusion to the spinal cord will result in a very rapid breakdown of the polyunsaturated fatty sheaths surrounding nerve pathways. Even a small bruise causes capillaries to leak blood. Erythrocytes are quickly caught up in a fibrin clot, causing hemolysis and release of free iron and copper. These metals act as potent catalysts which combine with oxygen to increase the rate of lipid peroxidation by a millionfold. Animal experiments show that this "chain reaction" can be squelched in at least two ways: (1) The spinal cord can be irrigated with a potent free radical scavenger such as dimethyl sulfoxide (DMSO) or (2) The iron and copper catalysts can be inactivated by bathing the injured area in a chelating solution containing EDTA or d-penicillamine.[70, 77, 108, 129–131] Hyperbaric oxygen can also halt free radical progression, retaining spinal cord and brain function. Both DMSO and hyperbaric oxygen are now being utilized in research protocols at major medical centers to prevent permanent paralysis in victims of spinal cord and brain injuries. Results thus far indicate that if treatment is begun within the first 30 minutes, or at most within the first two hours, the outcome is much better than would otherwise have been expected.[132–147]

Both chelation therapy and hyperbaric oxygen have been observed to alleviate or temporarily reverse the progression of multiple sclerosis (MS).[148, 149] MS victims experience degeneration of the polyunsaturated fatty insulating material of nerve pathways in the brain and spinal cord. Although free radical damage may be just one link in the chain of cause and effect, it is possible to slow the progress of this devastating disease in the majority of victims by using treatment principles which reduce free radical reactions.

TOBACCO AND ALCOHOL

It has long been known that habitual use of tobacco and excessive alcohol are related to illness and premature death. Alcohol causes damage and scarring of the liver and cancer in the mouth and digestive organs.[150]

Alcohol is metabolized to acetaldehyde, a free radical precursor. Acetaldehyde is closely related to formaldehyde (embalming fluid) which causes cross-linkages of connective tissue (tanning) by free radical reactions.[69, 70, 151, 152] Cirrhosis of the liver is quite literally a form of antemortem embalming.

Tobacco is associated with an increased incidence of atherosclerosis, cancer and other diseases. Tobacco contains polynuclear aromatic hydrocarbons which produce free radicals and free radical precursors in its combustion tars. These substances put a great strain on the body's free radical defenses and accelerate the onset of cancer, atherosclerosis and other degenerative conditions.[153] Processed tobacco contains cadmium, a heavy metal ten times more toxic than lead, which also acts as a catalyst of free radical reactions and actively competes with zinc in metalloactivated enzymes. Tobacco smoke also contains small amounts of radioactive isotopes which increase free radical damage from ionizating radiation.

CELL MEMBRANE METABOLISM

Every cell in the body is enveloped in a bipolar phospholipid membrane in which are suspended large enzyme molecules and other metabolically active components. This membrane has the characteristics of a viscous fluid and is constantly changing. It is relatively impermeable to substances which are not desired within the cell. The polar (water-soluble) ends of phospholipid molecules line the inner and outer surfaces of the cell membrane while the non-polar (fat soluble) tails point inward, traversing the interior of the cell wall. The normal cis- configuration of phospholipids causes them to coil around proteins and other molecular constituents within the membrane. This cis- curvature greatly influences the physical characteristics of the cell membrane and its associated enzyme activity.[66, 69, 70] Unoxidized cholesterol is widely disbursed within cell membranes and acts to protect against free radical damage. Oxidized dietary cholesterol which has been altered in food processing offers no such antioxidant protection. When free radicals approach a cell, cholesterol and a wide variety of other defenses normally prevent them from damaging the cell wall.

Large energy-dependent metabolic "pump" enzymes span the full thickness of cell membranes. They are bathed in plasma on the exterior and extend into the cytoplasm of the cell. One such pump maintains a higher concentration of sodium ions on the exterior of the cell wall and potassium on the interior. Another pump keeps a much higher concentration of calcium outside the cell and magnesium inside. Cellular organelles, including mitochrondria, lysosomes, endoplasmic reticuli and the Golgi mechanisms, are also enveloped in bipolar lipid membranes containing numerous energy-dependent transport mechanisms. The mitochondrial membrane contains coenzyme Q, necessary for energy production. Mitochondria are the power houses of cells and they normally produce free radicals during transport of electrons in the process of oxidative phosphorylation. Adequate antioxidant protection prevents these free radicals from proliferating.[66, 69, 70]

Receptor sites on cell membranes for neurotransmitters, insulin, and various other hormones are damaged by excessive free radicals. Calcium-magnesium and sodium-potassium pumps are impaired, allowing excessive calcium and sodium to enter cells. Free radicals damage nuclear membranes, altering nuclear pores and genetic material, causing impairment of protein synthesis and cell replication. Free radical mutations of DNA produce uncontrolled cell division and cancer. Free radicals increase the activity of guanylate cyclase which stimulates cell division. Lymphoid tissues are very rich in polyunsaturated fatty acids and free radical damage causes immunologic abnormalities. The immune system then attacks the body's own tissues in so-called autoimmune disease or it may be weakened and fail to recognize and destroy pathogenic organisms and malignant cells.[66, 69, 70, 74]

CALCIUM METABOLISM

Free radical impairment of the calcium-magnesium pump allows excessive calcium to enter the cell. Calcium activates phospholipase-A_2 which cleaves arachidonic acid from membrane phospholipids. Arachidonic acid then produces prostaglandins and leukotrienes, creating more free radicals in the process.[69, 70] Leukotrienes are potent inflammatory substances which attract leukocytes. Leukocytes, as we noted previously, produce superoxide free radicals during phagocytosis. Leukocytes out of control, excessively stimulated by leukotrienes, produce excessive free radicals and cause inflammatory damage to surrounding tissues.[69, 154] Small capillaries and arterioles dilate, causing edema, and leakage of erythrocytes through blood vessel walls. Platelets are stimulated to produce microthrombi. Erythrocytes hemolyze, releasing free copper and iron which catalyze a massive increase of peroxidative damage to adjacent tissues.

Excessive calcium in smooth muscle cells, caused by free radical damage to cell walls, is bound to calmodulin which activates myosin kinase, which in turn phosphorylates myosin. Myosin and actin then constrict, causing the muscle cell to shorten. Thus increased calcium within smooth muscle cells leads to spasm of the entire muscle. The same occurs in cells of the myocardium. When muscle fibers encircling arteries constrict, blood flow is reduced. Calcium channel blockers relieve symptoms by slowing abnormal entry of calcium into cells but they do not correct the underlying cause of the problem—free radical disruption of cell membranes.[69, 70, 155] Myocardial function is also impaired by excessive intracellular calcium, reducing the efficiency of oxygen utilization and placing an extra burden on an already impaired coronary artery system. If a coronary (or other) artery is partially occluded by atherosclerotic plaque, minor spasm may cause disabling symptoms. Myocardial infarction has been observed to occur as a result of pure spasm in a coronary artery which was completely free from plaque.[156] Unopposed thromboxane and serotonin are released by platelets in the presence of free radicals.[69, 70] Thromboxane and serotonin are both potent mediators of arterial spasm.

Intracellular calcium excesses result from a variety of other factors. Ionized plasma calcium, the metabolically active fraction not bound to protein, slowly increases with age, partially resulting from excessive dietary phosphates. The higher the concentration of ionized calcium outside a cell, the harder the calcium pump must work to prevent excessive calcium from leaking in. Nutritional calcium antagonists also slow calcium influx. These include dietary magnesium, manganese and potassium. Magnesium and manganese intakes are sub-optimal in the average American diet.[113] Potassium is rarely deficient, but an excessively high ratio of dietary sodium to potassium is common, causing sodium to leak into cells much like calcium, poisoning its metabolism in different ways. Further losses of potassium and magnesium caused by diuretic therapy may add to this problem.

The efficiency of energy metabolism is impaired by excessive stress. Stress increases circulating catecholamines which partially uncouple ATPase. Cells lose potassium and retain more calcium and sodium under stress because of this relative uncoupling of magnesium-calcium ATPase and sodium-potassium ATPase.

Catecholamines produce free radicals when they are metabolized.[69, 70] If the nervous system's free radical defenses have been exceeded, stress-related catecholamines cause free radical damage to neuronal receptors. This is one explanation for stress related nervous disorders. Metabolic degradation products of dopamine, a catecholamine neurotransmitter, can cause free radical damage to neuronal receptor sites in the brain, causing Parkinson's disease, and possibly some types of schizophrenia.[157] Neuronal receptors for norepinephrine can be damaged by free radicals, causing depression. Cardiac disease has also been shown to result from catecholamine induced free radical pathology.[158]

In recent animal experiments, primates subjected to stress were found to have an increased incidence of atherosclerosis, even while fed a diet otherwise protective against that disease. Increased free radical pathology associated with increased catecholamine metabolism could explain that finding.

Dementia of the Alzheimer's type is thought by some authorities to be the result of brain cell destruction by free radicals.[158] Arrest and improvement in a significant percentage of patients with Alzheimer's dementia has been reported following treatment with deferoxamine, an iron chelating agent.[159] Iron is a potent catalyst of lipid peroxidation. Accumulations of aluminum and lipid-protein breakdown pigments in areas of the brain affected by Parkinson's and Alzheimer's are now thought to be late events, not causative factors, much like the accumulation of calcium and cholesterol in arterial plaque.

Before the significance of free radical pathology became known, it was hypothesized that EDTA chelation therapy had its major effect on calcium metabolism. It is now apparent that calcium is just another link in the chain of cause and effect created by free radical damage. EDTA can influence calcium in many ways, but the calcium hypothesis was never adequate to explain the many benefits observed following chelation. Lack of an acceptable scientific explanation has greatly delayed more widespread acceptance.

EDTA lowers ionized plasma calcium during infusion. The body responds to maintain homeostasis with a dramatic increase in circulating parathormone.[160] The intermittent 3-4 hour pulses of increased parathormone caused by EDTA infusion have a profound effect on bone metabolism.[161] Frost's recently proposed concept of bone metabolism, known as the Basic Multicellular Unit (BMU) Theory, is now accepted by experts in this field.[162] The BMU theory helps to explain the causes and treatment of osteoporosis and osteopenia.

The BMU is a group of metabolically active cells which control the turn-over of approximately 0.1 mm^3 of bone tissue. When a BMU is activated it goes through a cycle consisting of an intial 3-4 weeks of bone absorption (osteoclastic phase) followed by a 2-3 month period of bone reformation (osteoblastic phase). Net increase or decrease in bone density at the end of the entire 3-4 month cycle depends on the rate and completeness of bone turnover, of nutritional adequacy and effective control of free radicals. Hormonal regulators of BMU's are thought to include growth hormone, thyroxin and adrenal corticosteroids, but parathormone remains the most important controlling factor.[161] Chronic parathormone excess has long been known to cause bone destruction. On the other hand, brief pulsatile increases in parathormone, which occur during intravenous EDTA chelation therapy, result in net new bone formation.[163]

Anabolic activation of BMU's by pulsatile parathormone provides a possible explanation for the delayed improvement seen in chelation patients. Pathologic calcium may be removed from arteries and other soft tissues for utilization in new bone formation. In their original studies, Meltzer and Kitchell reported treating 10 severely handicapped men with EDTA, all of whom suffered intractible angina. After approximately 20 infusions, therapy was discontinued because of initially disappointing results. Three months later, 9 out of 10 patients returned to report marked relief of angina (despite the absence of change in life style, smoking or nutritional habits).[7] This three-month delay in achieving full benefit has remained a consistent observation by chelating physicians over the years.

Post-menopausal women who are not supplemented with estrogen experience a great increase in circulating follicular stimulating hormone (FSH). Elevated FSH interferes with new bone formation by BMU cells and is regarded as a possible cause of post-menopausal osteoporosis.[164]

It was previously hypothesized that the removal of calcium from plaque and from undesirable cross-linkage sites could explain most of the benefits seen from chelation. But cross-linkages of other types, such as disulfide bonds caused by free radical reactions, are also important. EDTA can correct abnormal disulfide bridging and cross-linkages caused by calcium, lead, cadmium, aluminum and other toxic metals. An important benefit of chelation therapy can result from reduction of cross-linkages which improves elasticity of vascular walls and other tissues.[36, 37]

Vascular changes may not be seen arteriographically, in spite of significant clinical improvement. Using Poiseuille's Law of hemodynamics one can demonstrate that with perfect laminar flow, a mere 19% increase in the radius of a blood vessel will double the blood flow rate. In a vessel with a turbulent flow around an atherosclerotic plaque, this figure decreases to less than a 10% increase in diameter to cause a doubling of blood flow. In an organ with compromised circulation, an increase in blood flow of 10 to 20% could result in significant functional improvement and alleviation of ischemic symptoms. Changes in diameter of such small magnitude cannot be detected on arteriograms.

EDTA CHELATION THERAPY

EDTA can reduce the production of free radicals by a millionfold.[70, 165] It is not possible for free radical pathology to be catalytically accelerated by metallic ions in the presence of EDTA. Traces of unbound metallic catalysts must be present for uncontrolled proliferation of free radicals in living tissues. EDTA binds ionic metal catalysts, making them chemically inert and removing them from the body. Concentrations of metallic ions with the ability to catalyze lipid peroxidation are so tiny that even the traces remaining in distilled water can initiate such reactions.[70, 119]

Metallic ions with the ability to catalyze lipid peroxidation are those which readily change electrical valence by one unit. Two essential nutritional elements, iron and copper, are the most potent catalysts of lipid peroxidation. Catalytic iron and copper accumulate near phospholipid cell membranes in joint fluid and in cerebrospinal fluid with age and are released into tissue fluids following trauma or ischemia. These extracellular iron and copper ions have been shown to cause free radical tissue damage.[79, 87, 89, 91, 166-171]

TOXIC HEAVY METALS

EDTA has long been accepted as a treatment of choice for heavy metal poisoning. Toxic heavy metals affect metabolism in a variety of ways. Poisonous metals such as lead, mercury and cadmium react avidly with sulfur-containing amino acids on protein molecules. When lead reacts with sulfur on the cysteine or methionine moiety of a large protein molecule, enzyme activity is destroyed. Chelation therapy reactivates enzymes by removing toxic heavy metals. Concentrations of lead in human bones have increased more than 500-fold since the industrial revolution.[172] Bone lead is in equilibrium with other vital organs and tends to be released into the circulation under stress, increasing toxicity when it can least be tolerated.[173]

Lead takes on additional importance with respect to the antioxidant roles of glutathione and glutathione peroxidase. Lead reacts vigorously with sulfur-containing glutathione and completely neutralizes its ability to scavenge free radicals. As previously described, reduced glutathione is an essential antioxidant in the recycling of vitamins E, C, glutathione peroxidase, glutathione reductase and NADH. Lead therefore cripples the free radical scavenging activity of that entire protective array of antioxidants.

Lead reacts with selenium even more avidly than with sulfur, inactivating the selenium-containing enzyme, glutathione peroxidase. That enzyme neutralizes lipid peroxides in addition to its role in the antioxidant recycling system. Other toxic heavy metals also inactivate glutathione peroxidase. Multielement hair analysis is becoming accepted as a cost-effective screening test for heavy metal toxicity and as a method to screen for the nutritional status of some essential nutritional elements.[174-199] Definitive testing may then be more appropriately selected based on initial data from hair analysis.

The broad spectrum of benefits reported from EDTA chelation therapy can now be better understood. Copper and iron are not easily chelated by EDTA when tightly bound to metallo-activated enzymes and physiologic carrier molecules. On the other hand, when these nutritional elements accumulate in pathological locations which allow them to act as lipid peroxidation catalysts, they are quite readily removed by EDTA. Iron and copper both accumulate with age at pathological sites where they catalyze free radical damage.[34, 166-171] EDTA binds much more tightly to iron, copper and other free radical catalysts than it does to calcium. EDTA will only bind calcium if none of the other ions are readily available.[34] Although EDTA has become known as a calcium chelator, it is much more effective as a chelator of iron, copper and toxic heavy metals.

Iron accumulates more slowly in women during the child-bearing years because of monthly menstrual losses. Women in that age group also have significant protection against atherosclerosis which is lost at menopause. Body iron stores, as reflected by serum ferritin, confirm that men accumulate iron four times more rapidly than pre-menopausal women.[200] It is also notable that the risk of atherosclerosis is four times greater in men in this same age group. Data from the Framingham study documents immediate loss of protection and reversion of women to approximately the same relative risk of atherosclerosis as men following hysterectomy, even if the ovaries are not removed.[201 203] These observations provide evidence that slower iron accumulation rather than endocrine influence is responsible for reduced atherosclerosis in pre-menopausal women.[204] The fact that iron is a potent catalyst of lipid peroxidation provides a free radical explanation for these clinical and epidemiologic findings. EDTA has a high affinity for iron that is not already bound to hemoglobin or to a metalloenzyme.

The following lists the affinity of EDTA for various metals, at physiologic pH, in order of decreasing stability. In the presence of a more tightly bound metal, EDTA will drop a metal lower in the series and will chelate and remove the metal for which it has a greater affinity.[205] Calcium is near the bottom of the list while iron and copper are near the top.

chromium^{2+}
iron^{3+}
mercury^{2+}
copper^{2+}
lead^{2+}
zinc^{2+}
cadmium^{2+}
cobalt^{2+}
aluminum^{3+}
iron^{2+}
manganese^{2+}
calcium^{2+}
magnesium^{2+}

Magnesium is a calcium antagonist, desirable for most chelation patients, and is the metallic ion least likely to be removed by EDTA. In fact, EDTA is administered as magnesium-EDTA, providing an efficient delivery system to increase magnesium stores while simultaneously chelating other undesired metals.

The free radical benefits of EDTA explain the recently published observations of Blumer in Switzerland who reported a 90 percent reduction in deaths from cancer in a large group of chelation patients who had been carefully followed over an eighteen-year period. When compared with a statistically matched control group, Blumer reported a ten times greater death rate from cancer in the untreated group, compared to the chelation patients.[38] A greatly reduced incidence of cardiovascular deaths was also observed. The common denominator of both cancer and atherosclerosis is free radical pathology.[66, 69, 70] Blumer used calcium-EDTA which is assumed to have precluded any direct effect on calcium metabolism in these patients. Although he attributed benefits to lead removal, the patients studied had been exposed to the same environmental lead as an average resident in any large city. In light of the work of Demopoulos, chelation of free radical catalysts seems a more likely explanation. It was Demopoulos[89] who first proposed that chelation be used to control free radical pathology. Demopoulos also pointed out that many antioxidants have chelating properties.[66, 89]

EDTA increases the efficiency of mitochondrial oxidative phosphorylation and improves myocardial function, quite independently of any effect on arterial blood supply.[206] Treatment with deferoxamine, an iron chelator, has been shown to improve cardiac function in patients with thalassemia major.[207] Chelation with deferoxamine has also been shown to reduce inflammatory responses in animal experimentation.[208] Sullivan suggested that periodic donation of blood be studied as a means to reduce the risk of atherosclerosis in men and post-menopausal women.[204]

By interrupting the ongoing process of free radical damage, EDTA chelation therapy allows normal healing to proceed more rapidly than tissue destruction. This slow healing of damaged tissues is an explanation for the time lapse of several months following chelation before full benefit is observed. Stimulation of normal healing seems far superior to mere suppression of symptoms achieved with most other therapies.

CHELATION AND ATHEROSCLEROSIS

Let's look briefly at what is known about the cause of occlusive atherosclerotic cardiovascular disease. If an injury results in a cut artery, homeostatic mechanisms must quickly stop the flow of blood to prevent hemorrhage and death. This regulation of bleeding is under the control of a variety of mechanisms including extremely potent hormones called prostaglandins. Prostaglandins are produced and degraded continuously and very rapidly in the endothelium and platelets. Prostaglandins have a half-life measured in seconds and must be constantly synthesized in a proper balance to maintain normal blood flow.

The two important prostaglandins in relation to atherosclerosis are prostacyclin and thromboxane. Prostacyclin reduces the adhesiveness of platelets, allowing free flow of blood cells and plasma, reducing the tendency to fibrin deposition and thrombi. Prostacyclin relaxes encircling muscle fibers in artery walls, reducing spasm. Thromboxane does the opposite. It causes intense spasm in blood vessel walls and it stimulates platelets to adhere.[209] In over-simplified terms, thromboxane is the "bad guy" and prostacyclin is the "good guy." In actual fact, a proper balance must be maintained between the two to protect against injury and hemorrhage on the one hand and to maintain normal circulation on the other.

Synthesis of prostacyclin is completely blocked by the presence of lipid peroxides and free radicals while thromboxane remains unaffected. If lipid peroxides are present, either from dietary intake of excessive fats and oils, or from nearby peroxidation of lipoprotein cell membranes, no prostacyclin can be produced to balance the effects of thromboxane.[69, 70, 210]

Damage to vascular endothelium occurs routinely by direct free radical attack and from minor hemodynamic stresses related to normal blood flow and daily physical activity. Some such damage may be caused by a disordered immune system. Under healthy circumstances, minor vascular injuries are rapidly healed, aided by a thin layer of platelets which coat the disrupted surface with a protective blanket.[111] If free radical scavengers are inadequate and the local control threshold has been exceeded, the resulting proliferation of free radicals blocks the production of prostacyclin. Without prostacyclin, unopposed thromboxane causes the injured area of the arterial wall to become excessively attractive to platelets and platelets to become overly attracted to each other. Platelets rain down, building up an abnormally thick aggregation. This growing layer of platelets traps a number of leukocytes which also produce free radicals. A network of fibrin and microthrombi is formed and erythrocytes become trapped. Some of these erythrocytes hemolyze, causing free iron and copper to leak into the surrounding area. These metallic catalysts produce an explosive increase in free radical oxidation of cholesterol and phospholipid cell membranes. Prostacyclin production is increasingly inhibited for some distance along the blood vessel.

The resulting high concentrations of free radicals also damage nuclear material in one or more cells of the artery, causing mutation and loss of control of cell replication. Lipid peroxides increase the activity of guanylate cyclase, which speeds mitosis. This sequence of events eventually produces an atheroma, an enlarging tumor consisting of mutated, rapidly multiplying multi-potential cells which have lost their former high degree of differentiation and specialized functioning. Atheroma cells produce substantial amounts of connective tissue, collagen and elastin. They ingest cellular debris as macrophages. The monoclonal theory of atheroma formation first proposed by Benditt,[211] most accurately fits the known facts. Cholesterol is oxidized by free radical activity and some of the cholesterol oxidation products ingested by atheroma cells have vitamin D activity.[110]

Intracellular calcium is already abnormally high because of free radical damage to homeostatic mechanisms in cell walls. Localized excesses of vitamin D activity caused by oxidation of cholesterol produce further calcium accumulations. Calcium and cholesterol deposits accumulate in the late stages of atheroma formation. Increasing amounts of cholesterol are produced in an attempt to protect against free radical damage. Some is even produced within the atheroma.[212] Cholesterol is increasingly consumed by free radical oxidation. Oxidized cholesterol and cholesterol esters crystalize within the plaque. Eventually the plaque expands to exceed its own blood supply. When the interior of the plaque grows too far from the closest intact circulation to receive adequate oxygen and other nutrients, the central core of the plaque degenerates into an amorphous fibro-fatty mass which contains varying amounts of calcium, cholesterol, connective tissue and cellular debris. This necrotic core commonly ulcerates and embolizes. Ongoing free radical reactions continue to suppress prostacyclin causing a constant hailstorm of platelets. These platelets release high concentrations of thromboxane and serotonin, promoting arterial spasm which further occludes blood flow.

Symptoms begin to occur when a blood vessel becomes approximately 75 percent occluded. A large meal, rich in peroxidized fats, can cause a sudden additional free radical insult, triggering an abrupt increase in spasm or even an acute thrombosis.

Similar degenerative changes occur in all parts of the body. Cells swell and die as membranes become increasingly leaky and damaged. Active transport pumps become uncoupled or disabled. DNA damage results in mutation, increasing the probability of uncontrolled cell replication and cancer.[66] Lymphoid tissues and cells of the immune system become damaged.[69, 70, 74] Cross-linkages occur between connective tissue, elastin and enzymes molecules caused by free radical reactions and metallic ions. Tissues age rapidly and organ functions deteriorate. Joints become hypertrophic, inflamed and deformed. Leukotriene production and prostaglandin imbalances cause arthritis and inflammatory change in many organs. Lysosomes rupture, releasing proteolytic enzymes and devastating cell contents. Lysosomes have been called the cells' digestive organs and when disrupted lead to auto-digestion by cells. Free radicals react with available selenium, increasing the excretion of the resulting selenium compounds, creating a relative selenium deficiency. Cancer patients excrete selenium in amounts up to five times the normal rate, just when they need it the most.[113]

Antibody production and cellular immunity are increasingly impaired. Cells of the immune system are especially rich in polyunsaturated fats and are therefore highly vulnerable to free radical pathology. Oxidized cholesterol and lipid peroxides are potent immunosuppressants.[69, 74, 110] Foreign substances and malignant change, which would normally be disposed of, now overwhelm a weakened immunity which has lost its reserve. Partially digested food proteins which readily enter the circulation through the digestive tract are no longer tolerated.[213-215] Adverse reactions to specific foods (so-called "food allergies") develop. Free radical reactions, which occur normally within macrophages in the process of engulfing and destroying such foreign material, proceed out of control and cause tissue inflammation. Adverse tissue reactions to a variety of nutritious foods and other environmental exposures is a common occurrence. Avoidance of sensitizing foods and other triggering factors becomes necessary to control symptoms.[216-220] Potent antigenic properties of the common yeast, Candida albicans, normally present in the body in small numbers, now becomes overwhelming to the immune system. Candida organisms multiply more easily and produce potent toxins.[221-223] Yeast-related aspects of free radical disease become more prominent in a population raised on antibiotics, birth control pills, adrenocorticosteroids, and a diet high in refined carbohydrates—all of which stimulate excessive growth of Candida albicans.[224-227] A struggling immune system may become overreactive in other areas, attacking healthy tissues in so-called autoimmune states.

TREATMENT AND PREVENTION OF FREE RADICAL PATHOLOGY

The development of cancer often takes decades from the initiating event to the onset of symptoms. If cancer promoting factors are removed, free radical damage can be repaired and health can be restored by applied clinical nutrition and lifestyle corrections. Malignant cells in their early stages are able to undergo reverse transformation to a normal state. For example, smokers who stop the use of tobacco have the same risk of cancer ten years later as those who never smoked.[70] Atherosclerosis involves a non-malignant tumor, an atheroma, somewhat analagous to cancer. Free radical pathology is the common denominator. Atherosclerosis should also regress with time, if causative factors are corrected.

(1) Diet

Dietary fat and oil should be restricted to 20 percent or less of total calories.[69, 70] Consumption of fats and lipids which have been processed, extracted, exposed to air, heated, hydrogenated or in any way altered or removed from the food in which they naturally occur should be reduced as much as practical. Consumption of trace element-depleted refined carbohydrates (white flour, white rice, sugar) should be minimized. Total caloric intake should be moderated to maintain weight within at least 20 percent of ideal body weight. The use of salt should be restricted and no salt should be added at the table. Diets should contain ample amounts of fiber-rich whole grains and fresh vegetables. Very sick patients suffering with extensive free radical disease should be much stricter with diet until improvement occurs. Clinical improvement involves a healing process requiring months or years to complete.

(2) Nutritional Supplements

A scientifically balanced regimen of supplemental nutrients reinforces endogenous antioxidant defenses. Supplemental antioxidants and vitamins should include vitamins E, C, B_1, B_2, B_3, B_6, B_{12}, pantothenate, PABA, beta carotene and glutathione. A balanced program of mineral and trace element supplementation should include magnesium, zinc, selenium, manganese, and chromium. Trace elements can be toxic if taken to excess and supplemental copper and iron may speed free radical damage if not deficient. Iron and copper should be supplemented only to treat deficiency states diagnosed by serum ferritin and erythrocyte copper levels.[204, 228] Trace elements are essential to health and life but they can also cause harm. Trace element supplementation should be under the supervision of a health care professional who is knowledgeable in nutrition. Dietary histories and biochemical testing allow trace element supplementation to be tailored to the needs of each individual. Hair analysis is a cost effective screening test for copper deficiency and excess as well as evaluation of several other nutritional elements and accumulations of toxic heavy metals. Hair is not a reliable indicator of iron stores.[113, 174, 175, 229, 230]

(3) Moderating Health Destroying Habits

Tobacco: It is best to eliminate the use of tobacco altogether but, if that is not possible, a marked reduction in exposure would be helpful. This applies to cigarettes, pipe tobacco, cigars, snuff or chewing tobacco. Tobacco causes problems, even without combustion. Free radical precursors are absorbed from tobacco through the lining of the mouth and nose, even without inhaling smoke. A relatively healthy adult with adequate dietary intake of antioxidants may tolerate up to ten low-tar cigarettes (0.1 to 1 mg tar) per day without an increased risk of cancer. Even this amount increases the risk of atherosclerosis.[231]

Alcohol: Many victims of chronic degenerative diseases discover for themselves that alcohol is not well tolerated. For individuals with chronic illness complete avoidance may be advisable. A healthy adult should be able to tolerate and detoxify one to two ounces of pure ethanol per 24 hours (four eight-ounce glasses of beer, four small glasses of wine, or two to three shot glasses of hard liquor at most). That amount of alcohol can normally be consumed in 24 hours without exceeding the free radical control threshold.[69, 70]

(4) Physical Exercise

Moderate physical exercise, even a brisk 45-minute walk several times per week, will help to maintain efficient utilization of oxygen. More vigorous aerobic exercise results in proportionately greater benefits. Lactate accumulates in tissues up to twice normal levels with aerobic exercise, even a brisk walk.[232] Lactate has chelating properties and some benefits of exercise thought to result from chelation of undesired metallic elements.[37]

(5) Hyperbaric Oxygen

Intermittent exposures to 100 percent oxygen at up to twice normal atmospheric pressure can interrupt free radical pathology restoring the free radical control threshold in a variety of ways. Oxygen in proper controlled doses is an excellent free radical scavenger. Oxygen at reduced levels, as occurs in ischemic organs affected by atherosclerosis, causes free radical reactions to proceed more rapidly. Hyperbaric oxygen (HBO) raises oxygen tension in ischemic tissues to normal levels. HBO stimulates an adaptive increase in cellular levels of free radical scavenging enzymes such as superoxide dismutase.[118] Rebound dilatation of blood vessels occurs following HBO which improves blood flow to ischemic organs. HBO helps to kill disease causing organisms, especially anerobic bacteria, and stimulates the ingrowth of new blood vessels to ischemic areas. HBO protects the fatty insulating sheaths surrounding nerve tracts in the brain and spinal column from free radical damage, relieving symptoms of stroke, senility, multiple sclerosis and spinal cord injury. Hyperbaric oxygen is most effective in the early stages of these conditions.[121, 233]

(6) EDTA Chelation Therapy

By removing toxic heavy metals and abnormally situated iron

and copper with EDTA, even when present in only ultratrace amounts, the ongoing process of free radical damage from lipid peroxidation can be reduced by up to a million-fold. Other benefits occur from uncoupling of disulfide and metallic cross-linkages, by normalization of calcium metabolism, by reactivation of enzymes poisoned by lead and other toxic metals, and by restoration of normal prostacyclin production along blood vessel walls. Lasting benefits are possible with a series of intravenous EDTA infusions in conjunction with other preventive, nutritional and therapeutic measures.

The proper scientific application of EDTA chelation therapy, as endorsed by the American Board of Chelation Therapy,[234-236] should lead to rapid and widespread recognition and acceptance of this well-documented, safe and effective therapy.

REFERENCES

1. Clarke NE, Clarke CN, Mosher RE: The "in vivo" disolution of metastatic calcium: An approach to atherosclerosis. *Am J Med Sci* 1955;229:142–149.
2. Schroeder HA, Perry HM Jr: Antihypertensive effects of metal binding agents. *J Lab Clin Med* 1955;46:416.
3. Clarke NE, Clarke CN, Mosher RE: Treatment of angina pectoris with disodium ethylene diamine tetraacetic acid. *Am J Med Sci* 1956;232:654–666.
4. Boyle AJ, Casper JJ, McCormick H, *et al.*: Studies in human and induced atherosclerosis employing EDTA. (Swiss, Basel) *Bull Schweiz Akad Med Wiss* 1957;13:408.
5. Muller SA, Brunsting LA, Winkelmann RK: Treatment of scleroderma with a new chelating agent, edathamil. *Arch Dermatol* 1959;80:101.
6. Clarke NE Sr: Atherosclerosis, occlusive vascular disease and EDTA. *Am J Cardiol* 1960;6:233–236.
7. Meltzer LE, Ural ME, Kitchell JR: The treatment of coronary artery disease with disodium EDTA, in Seven MJ, Johnson, LA (eds): *Metal Binding in Medicine.* Philadelphia, J.B. Lippincott Co, 1960, pp 132–136.
8. Peters HA: Chelation therapy in acute, chronic and mixed

porphyria, in Seven MJ, Johnson LA (eds): *Metal Binding in Medicine.* Philadelphia, J.B. Lippincott Co, 1960, pp 190–199.

9. Seven MJ, Johnson LA (eds): *Metal Binding in Medicine: Proceedings of a Symposium Sponsored by Hahnemann Medical College and Hospital, Philadelphia.* Philadelphia, J.B. Lippincott Co, 1960.
10. Kitchell, JR, Meltzer LE, Seven MJ: Potential uses of chelation methods in the treatment of cardiovascular diseases. *Prog Cardiovasc Dis* 1961;3:338–349.
11. Peters HA: Trace minerals, chelating agents and the porphyrias. *Fed Proc* 1961;20(3) (Part II) (suppl 10):227–234.
12. Boyle AJ, Clarke NE, Mosher RE, McCann DS: Chelation therapy in circulatory and sclerosing diseases. *Fed Proc* 1961;20(3) (Part II) (suppl 10):243–257.
13. Soffer A, Toribara T, Sayman A: Myocardial responses to chelation. *Br Heart J* 1961 Nov; 23:690.
14. Peripheral Flow Opened Up. *Medical World News,* Mar 15, 1963;4:36–39.
15. Boyle AJ, Mosher RE, McCann DS: Some in vivo effects of chelation—I: Rheumatoid arthritis. *J Chronic Dis* 1963;16:325–328.
16. Aronov DM: First experience with the treatment of atherosclerosis patients with calcinosis of the arteries with trilon-B (disodium salt of EDTA). *Klin Med* (Russ, Moscow) 1963;41:19–23.
17. Soffer A, Chenoweth M, Eichhorn G, Rosoff B, Rubin M, Spencer H: *Chelation Therapy* Springfield, Illinois, Charles C. Thomas, 1964.
18. Soffer A: Chelation therapy for cardiovascular disease, in Soffer A (ed): *Chelation Therapy* Springfield, Illinois, Charles C. Thomas, 1964, pp 15–33.
19. Lamar CP: Chelation therapy of occlusive arteriosclerosis in diabetic patients. *Angiology* 1964;15:379–394.
20. Friedel W, Schulz FH, Schroder L: Therapy of atherosclerosis through mucopolysaccarides and EDTA (ethylene diamine tetraacetic acid). (German) *Deutsch Gesundh* 1965;20:1566–1570.
21. Lamar CP: Chelation endarterectomy for occlusive atherosclerosis. *J Am Geriatr Soc* 1966;14:272–293.

22. Birk RE, Rupe CE: The treatment of systemic sclerosis with EDTA, pyridoxine and reserpine. *Henry Ford Hospital Medical Bulletin* 1966 June;14:109–139.
23. Lamar CP: Calcium chelation of atherosclerosis, nine years' clinical experience. Read before the Fourteenth Annual Meeting of the American College of Angiology, San Juan, PR, Dec 8, 1968. (transcript available AAMP, 6151 West Century Blvd., #1114, Los Angeles, CA 90045).
24. Olwin JH, Koppel JL: Reduction of elevated plasma lipid levels in atherosclerosis following EDTA chelation therapy. *Proc Soc Exp Biol Med* 1968;128:1137–1139.
25. Leipzig LJ, Boyle AJ, McCann DS: Case histories of rheumatoid arthritis treated with sodium or magnesium EDTA. *J Chronic Dis* 1970;22:553–563.
26. Brücknerová O, Tuláček J: Chelates in the treatment of occlusive atherosclerosis. (Czech, Praha) *Vnitr Lek* 1972; 18:729–735.
27. Nikitina EK, Abramova MA: Treatment of atherosclerosis patients with Trilon-B (EDTA). (Russ, Moscow) *Kardiologiia* 1972;12:137–139.
28. Evers R: Chelation of vascular atheromatous disease. *Journal International Academy Metabology* 1972;2:51–53.
29. Kurliandchikov VN: Treatment of patients with coronary arteriosclerosis with unithiol in combination with vitamins. (Russ, Kiev) *Vrach Delo* 1973;6:8.
30. Zapadnick VI, *et al.*: Pharmacological activity of unithiol and its use in clinical practice. (Russ, Keiv) *Vrach Delo* 1973;8:122.
31. David O, Hoffman SP, Sverd J, Clark J, Voeller K: Lead and hyperactivity, behavioral response to chelation: A pilot study. *Am J Psychiatry* 1976;133:1155–1158.
32. Gordon GB, Vance RB: EDTA chelation therapy for atherosclerosis: History and mechanisms of action. *Osteopathic Annals* 1976;4:38–62.
33. Proceedings: Hearing on EDTA Chelation Therapy of the Ad Hoc Scientific Advisory Panel on Internal Medicine of the Scientific Board of the California Medical Society, March 26, 1976, San Francisco, California (transcript available AAMP, 6151 West Century Blvd., #1114, Los Angeles, CA 90045.
34. Halstead BW: *The Scientific Basis of EDTA Chelation Therapy.*

Colton, CA, 1979. Golden Quill Publishers, Box 1278, Colton, CA 92324, 1979.

35. Grumbles LA: Radionuclide studies of cerebral and cardiac circulation before and after chelation therapy. Read before the American Academy of Medical Preventics, Chicago, IL, May 27, 1979. (transcript available AAMP, 6151 West Century Blvd, #1114, Los Angeles, CA 90045)
36. Bjorksten J: The cross-linkage theory of aging as a predictive indicator. *Rejuvenation* 1980;8:59–66.
37. Bjorksten J: Possibilities and limitations of chelation as a means for life extension. *Rejuvenation* 1980;8:67–72.
38. Blumer W, Reich T: Leaded gasoline—a cause of cancer. *Environmental International* 1980;3:465–471.
39. Carpenter DG: Correction of biological aging. *Rejuvenation* 1980;8:31–49.
40. Casdorph HR: EDTA chelation therapy, efficacy in arterio-sclertic heart disease. *J Holistic Med* 1981;3(1):53–59.
41. Casdorph HR: EDTA chelation therapy II, efficacy in brain disorders. *J Holistic Med* 1981;3(2):101–117.
42. McDonagh EW, Rudolph CJ, Cheraskin E: An occulocerebro-vasculometric analysis of the improvement in arterial stenosis following EDTA chelation therapy. *J Holistic Med* 1982;4(1):21–23.
43. Olwin JH: EDTA Chelation Therapy. Read before the American Holistic Medical Association, University of Wisconsin, La Crosse, Wisconsin, May 28, 1981. (Available on audio cassette, AHMI, 6932 Little River Turnpike, Annandale, Virginia 22003).
44. McDonagh EW, Rudolph CJ, Cheraskin E: The influence of EDTA salts plus multivitamin-trace mineral therapy upon total serum cholesterol/high-density lipoprotein cholesterol. *Medical Hypothesis* 1982;9:643–646.
45. McDonagh EW, Rudolph CJ, Cheraskin E: The effect of intravenous disodium ethylenediaminetetraacetic acid (EDTA) upon blood cholesterol in a private practice environment. *Journal of the International Academy of Preventive Medicine* 1982;7:5–12.
46. Williams DR, Halstead BW: Chelating agents in medicine. *J Toxicol: Clin Toxicol* 1983;19(10):1081–1115.

47. Casdorph HR, Farr CH: EDTA chelation therapy III: Treatment of peripheral arterial occlusion, an alternative to amputation. *J Holistic Med* 1983;5(1):3–15.
48. Doolan PD, Schwartz SL, Hayes JR, Mullen JC, Cummings NB: An evaluation of the nephrotoxicity of ethylenediaminetetraacetate and diethylenetriaminepentaacetate in the rat. *Toxicol Appl Pharmacol* 1967;10:481–500.
49. Ahrens FA, Aronson AL: A comparative study of the toxic effects of calcium and chromium chelates of ethylenediaminetetraacetate in the dog. *Toxicol Appl Pharmacol* 1971;18:10–25.
50. Feldman EB: EDTA and angina pectoris. *Drug Therapy* 1975 Mar:62.
51. Wedeen RP, Mallik DK, Batuman V: Detection and treatment of occupational lead nephropathy. *Arch Intern Med* 1979;139:53–57.
52. Moel DI, Kuman K: Reversible nephrotoxic reactions to a combined 2, 3-dimercapto-1-propanol and calcium disodium ethylenediaminetetraacetic acid regimen in asymptomatic children with elevated blood levels. *Pediatrics* 1982;70(2):259–262.
53. McDonagh EW, Rudolph CJ, Cherskin E: The effect of EDTA chelation therapy plus supportive multivitamin-trace mineral supplementation upon renal function: A study in serum creatinine. *J Holistic Med* 1982;4:146–151.
54. Cranton EM: Kidney effects of ethylene diamine tetraacetic acid (EDTA): A literature review. *J Holistic Med* 1982;4:152–157.
55. Batuman V, Landy E, Maesaka JK, Wedeen RP: Contribution of lead to hypertension with renal impairment. *N Engl J Med* 1983; 309(1):17–21.
56. McDonagh EW, Rudolph CJ, Cheraskin E: The effect of EDTA chelation therapy plus supportive multivitamin-trace mineral supplementation upon rental function: A study in blood urea nitrogen (BUN). *J Holistic Med* 1983;5(2):(in press).
57. Kitchell JR, Palmon F, Aytan N, Meltzer LE: The treatment of coronary artery disease with disodium EDTA, a reappraisal. *Am J Cardiol* 1963;11:501–506.
58. Cranton EM, Frackelton JP: Current status of EDTA chela-

tion therapy in occlusive arterial disease. *J Holistic Med* 1982;4:24–33.

59. Wartman A, Lampe TL, McCann DS, Boyle AJ: Plaque reversal MgEDTA in experimental atherosclerosis: Elastin and collagen metabolism. *J Atheros Res* 1967;7:331.
60. Wissler RW: Principles of the pathogenesis of atherosclerosis, in Braunwald E (ed): *Heart Disease*. Philadelphia, W.B. Saunders Co, 1980, pp 1221–1236.
61. Kjeldsen K, Astrup P, Wanstrup J: Reversal of rabbit atherosclerosis by hyperoxia. *J Atheros Res* 1969;10:173.
62. Vesselinovitch D, Wissler RW, Fischer-Dzoga K, Hughes R, DuBien L: Regression of atherosclerosis in rabbits. I. Treatment with low fat diet, hyperoxia and hypolipidemic agents. *Atherosclerosis* 1974;19:259.
63. Sincock A: Life extension in the rotifer by application of chelating agents. *J Gerontol* 1975;30:289–293.
64. Wissler RW, Vesselinovitch D: Regression of atherosclerosis in experimental animals and man. *Mod Concepts Cardiovasc Dis* 1977;46:28.
65. Walker F: *The effects of EDTA chelation therapy on plaque, calcium, and mineral metabolism in arteriosclerotic rabbits,* Ph.D. thesis. Texas State University, 1980. (Available from University Microfilm International, Ann Arbor, MI 48016.)
66. Demopoulos HB, Pietronigro DD, Flamm ES, Seligman ML: The possible role of free radical reactions in carcinogenesis. *Journal of Environmental Pathology and Toxicology* 1980;3: 273–303.
67. Harman D: The aging process. *Proc Natl Acad Sci USA* 1981; 78:7124–7128.
68. Dormandy TL: An approach to free radicals. *Lancet* 1983;ii: 1010–1014.
69. Demopoulos HB, Peitronigro DD, Seligman ML: The development of secondary pathology with free radical reactions as a threshold mechanism. *Journal of the American College of Toxicology* 1983;2(3):173–184.
70. Demopoulos HB: Molecular oxygen in health and disease. Read before the American Academy of Medical Preventics 10th Annual Spring Conference, Los Angeles, CA, May 21, 1983.

(Available on 3 audio cassettes from Instatape, P.O. Box 1729, Monrovia, CA 91016.)
71. Ames BN: Dietary carcinogens and anticarcinogens. *Science* 1983;221:1256–1264.
72. Dormandy TL: Free-radical reaction in biological systems. *Ann R Coll Surg Engl* 1980;62:188–194.
73. Dormandy TL: Free-radical oxidation and antioxidants. *Lancet* 1978;i:647–650.
74. Levine SA; Reinhardt JH: Biochemical-pathology initiated by free radicals, oxidant chemicals, and therapeutic drugs in the etiology of chemical hypersensitivity disease. *J Orthomol Psychiatr* 1983;12(3):166–183.
75. Del Maestro RF: An approach to free radicals in medicine and biology. *Acta Physiol Scand* 1980;492(suppl):153–168.
76. Poole CP: *Electron Spin Resonance. A Comprehensive Treatise on Experimental Techniques.* New York, Interscience Publishers, 1967.
77. Demopoulos HB, Flamm ES, Seligman ML, Mitamura JA, Ransohoff J: Membrane perturbations in central nervous system injury: Theoretical basis for free radical damage and a review of the experimental data, in Popp AJ, Bourke LR, Nelson LR, Kimelbert HK (eds): *Neural Trauma*. New York, Raven Press, 1979, pp 63–78.
78. Seligman ML, Mitamura JA, Shera N, Demopoulos HB: Corticosteroid (methylprednisolone) modulation of photoperoxidation by ultraviolet light in liposomes. *Photochem Photobiol* 1979;29:549–558.
79. Pryor WA: Free radical reactions and their importance in biochemical systems. *Fed Proc* 1973;32:1862–1869.
80. Pryor WA (ed): *Free Radicals in Biology. Volumes 1-3.* New York, Academic Press, 1976.
81. Lambert L, Willis ED: The effect of dietary lipid peroxides, sterols and oxidised sterols on cytochrome P450 and oxidative demethylation. *Biochem Pharmacol* 1977a;26:1417–1421.
82. Lambert C, Willis ED: The effect of dietary lipids on 3, 4, benzo(a)pyrene metabolism in the hepatic endoplasmic reticulum. *Biochem Pharmcol* 1977b;26:1423–1477.
83. Fedorenko VI: Effect of cysteine, glutathione and 1-p-chloro-

phenyltetrazole-thione-2 on postradiation changes in the metabolic free radical content of albino rat tissues. *Radiobiologiia* 1979;19:67-73.
84. Fridovich I: Superoxide dismutases. *Annu Rev Biochem* 1975:147-159.
85. Black HS, Chan JT: Experimental ultraviolet light-carcinogenesis. *Photochem Photobiol* 1977;26:183-189.
86. Eaton GJ, Custer P, Crane R: Effects of ultraviolet light on nude mice: Cutaneous carcinogenesis and possible leukemogenesis. *Cancer* 1978;42:182-188.
87. Tappel AL: Lipid peroxidation damage to cell components. *Fed Proc* 1973;32:1870-1874.
88. Kotin P, Falk HL: Organic peroxides, hydrogen peroxide, epoxides and neoplasia. *Radiat Res* 1963;3(suppl):193-211.
89. Demopoulos, HB: Control of free radicals in the biologic systems. *Fed Proc* 1973;32:1903-1908.
90. Walling C: Forty years of free radicals, in Pryor WA (ed): *Organic Free Radicals*. Washington, DC, American Chemical Society, 1978.
91. Demopoulos HB: The basis of free radical pathology. *Fed Proc* 1973;32:1859-1861.
92. Tappel AL: Will antioxidant nutrients slow aging processes? *Geriatrics* 1968;23:97-105.
93. Coon MJ: Oxygen activation in the metabolism of lipids, drugs and carcinogens. *Nutr Rev,* 1978;36:319-328.
94. Coon MJ: Reconstitution of the cytochrome P-450-containing mixed-function oxidase system of liver microsomes. *Methods Enzymol* 1978a;52:200-206.
95. Coon MJ, van der Hoeven TA, Dahl SB, Haugen DA: Two forms of liver microsomal cytochrome P-450, P-4501m2 and P-450M4 (rabbit liver). *Methods Enzymol* 1978b;52:109-117.
96. Panganamala RV, Sharma HM, Sprecher H, Geer JC, Cornwell DG: A suggested role for hydrogen peroxide in the biosynthesis of prostaglandins. *Prostaglandins* 1974;8:3-11.
97. Maisin JR, Décleve A, Gerber GB, Mattelin G, Lambiet-Collier M: Chemical protection against the long-term effects of a single whole-body exposure of mice to ionizing radiation. II. Causes of death. *Radiat Res* 1978;74:415-435.

NT: In vivo evidence for superoxide and peroxide production by adriamycin and cis- platium, Autor A (ed) *Active Oxygen and Medicine.* New York, Raven Press, 1980.
99. Petkau A: Radiation protection by superoxide dismutase. *Photochem Photobiol* 1978;28:765–774.
100. Schaefer A, Komlos M, Seregi A: Lipid peroxidation as the cause of the ascorbic acid induced decrease of ATPase activities of rat brain microsomes and its inhibition by biogenic amines and psychotropic drugs. *Biochem Pharmcol* 1975;24: 1781–1786.
101. Vladimirov YA, Sergeer PV, Seifulla RD, Rudnev YN: Effect of steroids on lipid peroxidation and liver mitochondrial membranes: *Molekuliarnaia Biologiia* (Russ, Moscow) 1973; 7: 247–262. (Translated by Consultants Bureau, a division of Plenum Publishing Inc, New York, New York.)
102. Sies H, Summer KH: Hydroperoxide-metabolizing systems in rat liver. *Eur J Biochem* 1975;57:503–512.
103. Alfthan G, Pikkarainen J, Huttunen JK, Puska P: Association between cardiovascular death and myocardial infarction and serum selenium in a matched-pair longitudinal study. *Lancet* 1982;2(8291):175–179.
104. Willett WC, Morris JS, Pressel S, *et al.*: Prediagnostic serum selenium and risk of cancer. *Lancet* 1983;2(8343):130–134.
105. Demopoulos HB, Flamm ES, Seligman ML, Jorgensen E, Ransohoff J: Antioxidant effects of barbiturates in model membranes undergoing free radical damage. *Acta Neurol Scand* 1977;56(suppl 64):152.
106. Flamm ES, Demopoulos HB, Seligman ML, Mitamura JA, Ransohoff J: Barbiturates and free radicals, in Popp AJ, Popp RS, Bourke LR, Nelson, Kimelberg HK (eds): *Neural Trauma.* New York, Raven Press, 1979, pp 289–300.
107. Butterfield JD; McGraw CP: Free radical pathology. *Stroke* 1978;9(5):443–445.
108. Demopoulos HB, Flamm ES, Pietronigro DD, Seligman ML: The free radical pathology and the microcirculation in the major central nervous system disorders. *Acta Physiol Scand* 1980;492(suppl):91–119.

109. Seligman ML, Demopoulos HB: Spin-probe analysis of membrane perturbations produced by chemical and physical agents. *Ann NY Acad Sci* 1973;222:640–667.
110. Smith LL: *Cholesterol Autooxidation.* New York, Plenum Press, 1981.
111. Gaby AR: Nutritional factors in cardiovascular disease. *J Holistic Med* 1983;5(2):(in press).
112. Taylor CB, Peng SK, Werthessen NT, Tham P, Lee KT: Spontaneously occurring angiotoxic derivatives of cholesterol. *Am J Clin Nutr* 1979;32:40.
113. Passwater RA, Cranton EM: *Trace Elements, Hair Analysis and Nutrition* New Canaan, CT, Keats Publishing, Inc, 1983.
114. Fourcans B: Role of phospholipids in transport and enzymic reactions. *Adv Lipid Res* 1974:147–226.
115. Babior BM: Oxygen-dependent microbial killing by phagocytes. *N Engl J Med* 1978;298:659–668.
116. Rosen H, Klebanoff SJ: Bactericidal activity of a superoxide anion-generating system. *J Exp Med* 1979;149:27–39.
117. Masterson WL, Slowinski E: In *Chemical Principles.* Philadelphia, Saunders, 1977, p 203, plate 5.
118. Mayes PA: Biologic oxidation, in Martin DW, Mayes PA, Rodwell VW (eds): *Harper's Review of Biochemistry.* Los Alton, CA, Lange Medical Publications, 1983, pp 129–130.
119. March J: *Advanced Organic Chemistry Reactions, Mechanics, and Structure,* ed. 2. New York, McGraw-Hill, 1978, p 620.
120. Flamm ES, Demopoulos HB, Seligman ML, Poser RG, Ransohoff J: Free radicals in cerebral ischemia. *Stroke* 1978;9(5): 445–447.
121. Hyperbaric Oxygen Therapy: A Committee Report, February 1981. Undersea Medical Society, Inc., 9650 Rockville Pike, Bethesda, Maryland 20014 (UMS Publication Number 30 CR(HBO) 2-23-81).
122. Foote CS: Chemistry of singlet oxygen VII. Quenching by beta carotene. *J Am Chem Soc* 1968;90:6233.
123. Peto R, Doll R, Buckley JD, Sporn MB: Can dietary beta-carotene materially reduce human cancer rates? *Nature* 1981;290:201.
124. Schaefer A, Komlos M, Seregi A: Lipid peroxidation as the

cause of the ascorbic acid induced decrease of ATPase activities of rat brain microsomes and its inhibition by biogenic amines and psychotropic drugs. *Biochem Pharmacol* 1975;24: 1781–1786.
125. Ito T, Allen N, Yashon D: A mitochondrial lesion in experimental spinal cord trauma. *J Neurosurg* 1978;48:434–442.
126. Atherosclerosis and auto-oxidation of cholesterol, editorial. *Lancet* 1980;ii:964–965.
127. Pietronigro DD, Demopoulos HB, Hovsepian M, Flamm ES: Brain ascorbic acid (AA) depletion during cerebral ischemia. *Stroke* 1982;13(1):117.
128. Demopoulos HB, Flamm ES, Seligman ML, Pietronigro DD, Tomasula T, DeCrescito V: Further studies on free-radical pathology in the major central nervous system disorders: effect of very high doses of methylprednisolone on the functional outcome; morphology, and chemistry of experimental spinal cord impact injury. *Can J Physiol Pharmacol* 1982;60 (11):1415–1424.
129. Flamm ES, Demopoulos HB, Seligman ML, Poser RG, Ransohoff J: Free radicals in cerebral ischemia. *Stroke* 1978;9:445.
130. Demopoulos HB, Flamm ES, Seligman ML, Pietronigro DD: Oxygen free radicals in central nervous system ischemia and trauma, in Autor AP (ed): *Pathology of Oxygen*. New York, Academic Press, 1982, pp 127–155.
131. Demopoulos HB, Flamm ES, Seligman ML, Ransohoff J: Molecular pathogenesis of spinal cord degeneration after traumatic injury, in Naftchi NE (ed): *Spinal Cord Injury*. New York & London, Spectrum Publications, Inc, 1982, pp 45–64.
132. Sukoff MH, Hollin SA, Espinosa OE, *et al.*: The protective effect of hyperbaric oxygenation in experimental cerebral edema. *J Neurosurg* 1968;29:236–239.
133. Kelly DL Jr, Lassiter KRL, Vongsvivut A, *et al.*: Effects of hyperbaric oxygen and tissue oxygen studies in experimental paraplegia. *J Neurosurg* 1972;36:425–429.
134. Holbach KH, Wassman H, Hoheluchter KL, *et al.*: Clinical course of spinal lesions treated with hyperbaric oxygen. *Acta Neurochir* 1975;31:297–298.
135. Holbach KH, Wassman H, Linke D: The use of hyperbaric

oxygenation in the treatment of spinal cord lesions. *Eur Neurol* 1977;16:213–221.
136. Yeo JD, Stabback S, McKinsey B: Study of the effects of hyperbaric oxygenation on experimental spinal cord injury. *Med J Aust* 1977;2:145–147.
137. Jones RF, Unsworth IP, Marasszeky JE: Hyperbaric oxygen and acute spinal cord injuries in humans. *Med J Aust* 1978;2:573–575.
138. Yeo JD, Lawry C: Preliminary report on ten patients with spinal cord injuries treated with hyperbaric oxygenation. *Med J Aust* 1978;2:572–573.
139. Gelderd JB, Welch DW, Fife WP, *et al.*: Therapeutic effects of hyperbaric oxygen and dimethyl sulfoxide following spinal cord transections in rats. *Undersea Biomedical Research* 1980;7:305–320.
140. Sukoff MH: Central nervous system: Review and update cerebral edema and spinal cord injuries. *HBO Review* 1980;1: 189–195.
141. Jesus-Greenberg DA: Acute spinal cord injury and hyperbaric oxygen therapy: A new adjunct in management. *Journal of Neurosurgical Nursing* 1980;12:155–160.
142. Higgins AC, Pearlstein MS, Mullen JB, *et al.*: Effects of hyperbaric oxygen therapy on long-tract neuronal conduction in the acute phase of spinal cord injury. *J Neurosurg* 1981;55(4): 501–510.
143. Sukoff MH, Ragatz RE: Use of hyperbaric oxygen for acute cerebral edema *Neurosurgery* 1982;10:29–38.
144. De La Torre JC, Johnson CM, Goode DJ, Mullan S: Pharmacologic treatment and evaluation of permanent experimental spinal cord trauma. *Neurology* 1975;25:508–514.
145. De La Torre JC, Kawanaga HM, Rowed DW, *et al.*: Dimethyl sulfoxide in central nervous system trauma. *Ann NY Acad Sci* 1975,243:362–389.
146. De La Torre JC, Surgeon JW: Dexamethasone and DMSO in experimental transorbital cerebral infarction. *Stroke* 1976;7: 577–583.
147. Laha RK, Dujovny M, Barrioneuvo PJ, *et al.*: Protective effects of methyl prednisolone and dimethyl sulfoxide in experi-

mental middle cerebral artery embolectomy. *J Neurosurg* 1978;49:508–516.

148. Fischer BH, Marks M, Reich T: Hyperbaric-oxygen treatment of multiple sclerosis. *N Engl J Med* 1983;308:181–186.

149. Swank R: *A Biochemical Basis of Multiple Sclerosis*. Springfield, IL, Charles C. Thomas, 1961.

150. Cimino JA, Demopoulos HB: Introduction: Determinants of cancer relevant to prevention, in the war on cancer. *Journal of Environmental Pathology and Toxicology* 1980;3:1–10.

151. Seligman ML, Flamm ES, Goldstein BD, Poser RG, Demopoulos HB, Ransohoff J: Spectrofluorescent detection of malonaldehyde as a measure of lipid free radical damage in response to ethanol potentiation of spinal cord trauma. *Lipids* 1977;12(11):-945–950.

152. Flamm ES, Demopoulos HB, Seligman ML, Tomasula JJ, DeCrescito V, Ransohoff J: Ethanol potentiation of central nervous system trauma. *J Neurosurg* 1977;46:328–334.

153. Dix T: Metabolism of polycyclic aromatic hydrocarbon derivatives to ultimate carcinogens during lipid peroxidation. *Science* 1983;221:77.

154. Samuelsson B: Leukotrienes: Mediators of immediate hypersensitivity reactions and inflammation. *Science* 1983;220: 568–575.

155. Hess ML, Manson NH; Okabe E: Involvement of free radicals in the pathophysiology of ischemic heart disease. *Can J Physiol Pharmacol* 1982;60(11):1382–1389.

156. Vincent GM, Anderson JL, Marshall HW: Coronary spasm producing coronary thrombosis and myocardial infarction. *N Engl J Med* 1983;309(14):220–239.

157. Harmon D: The free radical theory of aging. Read before the Orthomolecular Medical Society, San Francisco, CA, May 8, 1983. (Available on audio cassette from AUDIO-STATS, 3221 Carter Avenue, Marina Del Rey, CA 90291.)

158. Singal PK, Kapur N, Dhillon KS, Beamish RE, Dhalla NS: Role of free radicals in catecholamine-induced cardiomyopathy. *Can J Physiol Pharmacol* 1982;60(11):1340–1397.

159. Crapper-McLaughlin DR: Aluminum Toxicity in senile dementia: Implications for treatment. Read before the Fall Con-

ference, American Academy of Medical Preventics, Las Vegas, NV, Nov 8, 1981. (Available on audio cassette from AAMP, 6151 West Century Blvd., #1114, Los Angeles, CA 90045.)

160. Raymond JP, Merceron R, Isaac R, Wahbe F: Effects of EDTA and hypercalcemia on plasma prolactin, parathyroid hormone and calcitonic in normal and parathyroidectomized individuals. Read before the Frances and Anthony D'Anna International Memorial Symposium, Clinical Disorders of Bone and Mineral Metabolism, May 8, 1983. (Abstract available from Henry Ford Hospital, Dearborn, Michigan.)
161. Frost HB: Coherence treatment of osteoporosis. *Orthop Clin North Am* 1981;12:649–669.
162. DeLuca HF, Frost HM, Jee WSS, *et al.* (eds): *Osteoporosis: Recent Advances in Pathogenesis and Treatment.* Baltimore, University Park Press, 1981.
163. Frost HM: Treatment of osteoporosis by manipulation of coherent bone cell populations. *Clin Orthop* 1979;143:227–244.
164. Meyer MS, Chalmers TM, Reynolds JJ: Inhibitory effect of follicular stimulating hormone in parathormone in rat calvaria in vitro. Read before the Frances and Anthony D'Anna International Memorial Symposium, Clinical Disorders of Bone and Mineral Metabolism, May 8, 1983. (Abstract available from Henry Ford Hospital, Dearborn, Michigan.)
165. Wills ED: Lipid peroxide formation in microsomes. *Biochem J* 1969;113:325–332.
166. Gutteridge JMC, Rowley DA, Halliwell B, Westermarck T: Increased non-protein-bound iron and decreased protection against superoxide-radical damage in cerebrospinal fluid from patients with neuronal ceroid lipofuscinoses. *Lancet* 1982;ii: 459–460.
167. Willson RL: Iron, zinc, free radicals and oxygen tissue disorders and cancer control, In Iron Metabolism. *Ciba Foundn Symp 51* (new series). Amsterdam: Elsevier, 1977, pp 331–354.
168. Gutteridge JMC: Fate of oxygen free radicals in extracellular fluid. *Biochem Soc Trans* 1982;10:72–74.
169. Wills ED: Mechanisms of lipid peroxide formation in tissues: Role of metals and haematin proteins in the catalysis of the oxidation of unsaturated fatty acids. *Biochem Biophys Acta* 1965;98:238–251.

170. Gutteridge JMC, Rowley DA, Halliwell B: Superoxide-dependent formation of hydroxyl radicals and lipid peroxidation in the presence of iron salts. *Biochem J* 1982;206:605–609.
171. Heys AD, Dormandy TL: Lipid peroxidation in iron-overloaded spleens. *Clinical Science* 1981;60:295–301.
172. Ericson JE, Shirahata H, Patterson CC: Skeletal concentrations of lead in ancient Peruvians. *N Engl J Med* 1979;300:946–951.
173. Schroder HA: *The Poisons Around Us.* Bloomington, IN, Indiana University Press, 1974, p 49.
174. Jenkins DW: *Toxic Trace Metals in Mammalian Hair and Nails.* US Environmental Protection Agency publication No. (EPA)-600/4-79-049. Environmental Monitoring Systems Laboratory, 1979.
175. Cranton EM, Bland JS, Chatt A, Krakovitz R, Wright JV: Standardization and interpretation of human hair for elemental concentrations. *J Holistic Med* 1982;4:10–20.
176. Hansen JC, Christensen LB, Tarp U: Hair lead concentration in children with minimal cerebral dysfunction. *Danish Med Bull* 1980;27:259–262.
177. Medeiros DM, Pellum LK, Brown BJ: The association of selected hair minerals and anthropometric factors with blood pressure in a normotensive adult population. *Nutr Research* 1983;3:51–60.
178. Moser PB, Krebs NK, Blyler E: Zinc hair concentrations and estimated zinc intakes of functionally delayed normal sized and small-for-age children. *Nutr Research* 1982;2:585–590.
179. Thimaya S, Ganapathy SN: Selenium in human hair in relation to age, diet, pathological condition and serum levels. *Sci Total Environ* 1982;24:41–49.
180. Musa-Alzubaidi L, Lombeck I, Kasperek K, Feinendegen LE, Bremer HJ: Hair selenium content during infancy and childhood. *Eur J Pediatr* 1982;139:295–296.
181. Gibson RS, Gage L: Changes in hair arsenic levels in breast and bottle fed infants during the first year of infancy. *Sci Total Environ* 1982;26:33–40.
182. Ely DL, Mostardi RA, Woebkenberg N, Worstell D: Aerometric and hair trace metal content in learning-disabled children. *Environ Res* 1981;25(2):325–339.

183. Yokel RA: Hair as an indicator of excessive aluminum exposure. *Clin Chem* 1982;28(4):662–665.
184. Bhat RK, *et al.*: Trace elements in hair and environmental exposure. *Sci Total Environ* 1982;22(2):169–178.
185. Hurry VJ, Gibson RS: The zinc, copper, and manganese status of children with malabsorption syndromes and inborn errors of metabolism. *Biol Trace Element Res* 1982;4:157–173.
186. Thatcher RW, Lester ML, McAlester R, Horst R: Effects of low levels of cadmium and lead on cognitive functioning in children. *Arch Environ Health* 1982;37(3):159–166.
187. Peters HA, Croft WA, Woolson EA, Darcey BA: Arsenic, chromium, and copper poisoning from burning treated wood. *N Engl J Med* 1983;308(22):1360–1361.
188. Yamanaka S, Tanaka H, Nishimura M: Exposure of Japanese dental workers to mercury. *Bull Tokyo Den Coll* 1982;23:15–24
189. Capel ID, Spencer EP, Levitt HN, Daivies AE: Assessment of zinc status by the zinc tolerance test in various groups of patients. *Clin Biochem* 1982;15(2):257–260.
190. Vanderhoff JA, *et al.*: Hair and plasma zinc levels following exclusion of biliopancreatic secretions from functioning gastrointestinal tract in humans. *Dig Dis Sci* 1983;28(4):300–305.
191. Foli MR, Hennigan C, Errera J: A comparison of five toxic metals among rural and urban children. *Environ Pollut Ser A Ecol Biol* 1982;29:261–270.
192. Collipp PJ, Kuo B, Castro-Magana M, Chen SY, Salvatore S Hair zinc levels in infants. *Clin Pediatr* 1983;22(7):512–513.
193. Medeiros DM, Borgman RF: Blood pressure in young adults as associated with dietary habits, body conformation, and hair element concentrations. *Nutr Res* 1982;2:455–466.
194. Huel G, Boudene C, Ibrahim MA: Cadmium and lead content of maternal and newborn hair: Relationship to parity, birth weight, and hypertension. *Arch Environ Health* 1981;35(5) 221–227.
195. Marlowe M, Folio R, Hall D, Errera J: Increased lead burdens and trace mineral status in mentally retarded children. *J Spe Educ* 1982;16:87–99.
196. Marlowe M, Errera J, Stellern J, Beck D: Lead and mercury levels in emotionally disturbed children. *J Orthomol Psychiat* 1983; 12(4):260–267.

197. Nolan KR: Copper toxicity syndrome. *J Orthomol Psychiatr* 1983;12(4):270–282.
198. Klevay L: Hair as a biopsy material—assessment of copper nutriture. *Am J Clin Nutr* 1970;23(8):1194–1202.
199. Rees EL: Aluminum poisoning of papua New Guinea natives as shown by hair testing. *J Orthomol Psychiatr* 1983;12(4): 312–313.
200. Cook JD, Finch CA, Smith NJ: Evaluation of the iron status of a population. *Blood* 1976;48:449–455.
201. Kannel WB, Hjortland MC, McNamara PM, Gordon T: Menopause and the risk of cardiovascular disease. The Framingham Study. *Ann Intern Med* 1976;85:447–452.
202. Hjortland MC, McNamara PM, Kannel WB: Some atherogenic concomitants of menopause: The Framingham Study. *Am J Emidemiol* 1976;103:304–311.
203. Gordon T, Kannel WB, Hjortland MC, McNamara PM: Menopause and coronary heart disease. The Framingham Study. *Ann Intern Med* 1978;89:157–161.
204. Sullivan JL: Iron and the sex difference in heart disease risk. *Lancet* 1981;1(8233):1293–1294.
205. Skoog DA, West DM: Volumetric methods based on complexformation reactions, in *Fundamentals of analytical chemistry* New York, Holt, Rinehart and Winston, Inc, 1969, pp 338–360.
206. Peng CF, Kane JJ, Murphy ML, Straub KD: Abnormal mitochondrial oxidative phosphorylation of ischemic myocardium reversed by calcium chelating agents. *J Mol Cel Cardiol* 1977;9:897–908.
207. Freeman AP, Giles RW, Berdoukas VA, Walsh WF, Choy D, Murray PC: Early left ventricular dysfunction and chelation therapy in thalassemia major. *Ann Intern Med* 1983;99: 450–454.
208. Blake DR, Hall ND, Bacon PA, Dieppe PA, Halliwell B, Gutteridge JMC: Effect of a specific iron chelating agent on animal models of inflammation. *Ann Rheum Dis* 1983;42:89–93.
209. Addonizo VP, Wetstein L, Fisher CA, Feldman P, Strauss JF, Harken AH: Mediation of cardiac ischemia by thromboxanes released from human platelets. *Surgery* 1982;92:292.
210. Yagi K, Ohkawa H, Ohishi N, Yamashita M, Nakashima T: Lesion of aortic intima caused by intravenous administration

of linoleic acid hyperoxide. *J Appl Biochem* 1981;3:58–65.
211. Benditt EP: The origin of atherosclerosis. *Scientific American* Feb 1977, pp 74–85.
212. McCullach KG: Revised concepts of atherogenesis. *Cleve Clin Q* 1976;43:247.
213. Mayron LW: Portals of entry—a review. *Ann Allerg* 1978;40: 399–405.
214. Walker WA, Isselbacher KJ: Uptake and transport of macromolecules by the intestine: Possible role in clinical disorders. *Gastroenterology* 1974;67:531–550.
215. Hemmings WA, Williams EW: Transport of large breakdown products of dietary protein through the gut wall. *Gut* 1978;19:715–723.
216. Rowe AH, Rowe AH Jr: *Food Allergy: Its Manifestations and Control and the Elimination Diets.* Springfield, IL, Charles C. Thomas, 1972.
217. Speer F (ed): *Allergy of the Nervous System.* Springfield, IL, Charles C. Thomas, 1970.
218. Dickey LD (ed): *Clinical Ecology.* Springfield, IL, Charles C. Thomas, 1976.
219. Randolph TG: *Human Ecology and Susceptibility to the Chemical Environment* Springfield IL, Charles C. Thomas, 1962.
220. Crook WG: The coming revolution in medicine. *J Tenn Med Assn* 1983;76(3):145–149.
221. Iwata K: Toxins produced by Candida albicans. *Contr Microbiology Immunol* 1977;4:77–85.
222. Iwata K, Yamamota Y: Glycoprotein toxins produced by Candida albicans. Reprinted from Proceedings of the Fourth International Conference on the Mycoses. *PAHO Scientific Publication* 1977;356:246–257.
223. Iwata K: Fungal toxins as a parasitic factor responsible for the establishment of fungal infections. *Mycopathologia*; 65:141–154.
224. Crook WG: The Yeast Connection: *A Medical Breathrough.* Jackson, TN, Professional Books, 1984 (P.O. Box 3494, Jackson, TN 38301).
225. Truss CO: Tissue injury induced by candida albicans. *Orthomolecular Psychiatry* 1978;7(1):17–37.

226. Truss CO: Restoration of immunologic competence to candida albicans. *Orthomolecular Psychiatry* 1980;9(4):287–301.
227. Truss CO: The role of candida albicans in human illness. *Orthomolecular Psychiatry* 1981;10(4):228–238.
228. Hatano S, Nishi Y, Usui T: Copper levels in plasma and erythrocytes in healthy Japanese children and adults. *Am J Clin Nutr* 1982;35:120–126.
229. Harrison W, Yurachek J, Benson C: The determination of trace elements in human hair by atomic absorption spectroscopy. *Clin Chim Acta* 1969;23(1):83–91.
230. Klevay L: Hair as a biopsy material—assessment of copper nutriture. *Am J Clin Nutr* 1970;23(8):1194–1202.
231. Glori GB: Observed no-effect thresholds and the definition of less hazardous cigarettes. *Journal of Environmental Pathology and Toxicology* 1980;3:193–203.
232. Saltin B, Karlsson J: *Muscle Metabolism During Exercise.* New York, Plenum Publishing Co, 1971, p 395.
233. de Jesus-Greenberg D: Hyperbaric oxygen therapy. *Critical Care Update* 1981;8(2):8–20.
234. Important Facts You Should Know About The American Board of Chelation Therapy, 1983. American Board of Chelation Therapy, 1312 N.W. 12th Street, Moore, Oklahoma 73170.
235. American Board of Chelation Therapy. Constitution and By-Laws, April 1983. American Board of Chelation Therapy, 1312 N.W. 12th Street, Moore, Oklahoma 73170.
236. Protocol for the Safe and Effective Use of EDTA Chelation Therapy, 1983. American Board of Chelation Therapy, 1312 N.W. 12th Street, Moore, Oklahoma 73170.

Index

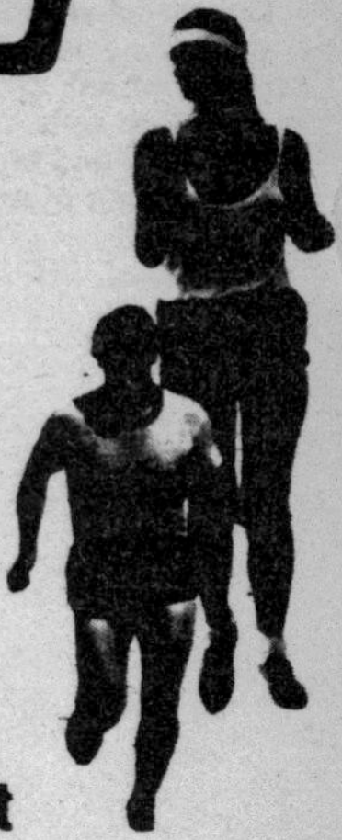

THE OFFICIAL EATING TO WIN COOKBOOK

Sports nutrition is an idea whose time has come. Author Frances Goulart's *The Official Eating to Win Cookbook*, a companion volume to her original book on sports nutrition, *Eating to Win*, tells weekend athletes how to select and prepare the foods that will give them that "extra edge" in their sport. It teaches the principles of an eating-to-win diet and provides over 200 easy-to-prepare recipes for the athlete: breakfasts, soups, salads, main dishes, desserts, snacks, drinks, and liquid meals.